Clinical Education in Geriatrics

This book highlights both recent innovations in professional health curricula and continuing education and interventions aimed at improving student attitudes towards geriatrics and aging.

The contributors cover areas including simulation, online training, and standardized patients for evaluation, but also emphasize the important end-result of clinical training: to take care of real older adults outside the classroom. Importantly, this underscores the development of powerful learning experiences of students by sensitizing them to the frameworks of palliative care, cancer care, sexuality, and aging research, all of which serves as a powerful catalyst for creating a 'pipeline' of students who embrace aging as a central theme of their future work.

As increased training in geriatrics is required to attune the health-care workforce to the needs of older adults, this book will be of interest to those seeking to create a more age-friendly health-care curriculum.

This book was originally published as a special issue of the *Gerontology & Geriatrics Education* journal.

Judith L. Howe is a Professor of Geriatrics and Palliative Medicine at the Icahn School of Medicine at Mount Sinai as well as Associate Director/Education and Evaluation at the James J. Peters VAMC Geriatrics Research, Education and Clinical Center, New York City, USA. She is also the Editor-in-Chief of *Gerontology and Geriatrics Education*. Dr. Howe has directed a number of interprofessional education and training programs and has served in national leadership positions in the field of gerontological education.

Thomas V. Caprio is a Professor of Medicine, Geriatrics, Dentistry, Clinical Nursing, and Public Health Sciences at the University of Rochester Medical Center, New York, USA. He is the Director of the Finger Lakes Geriatrics Education Center, has served in national leadership positions in geriatrics education, and is the Associate Editor for Clinical Education in Geriatrics for *Gerontology and Geriatrics Education*.

Clinical Education in Geriatrics

Innovative and Trusted Approaches Leading
Workforce Transformation in Making
Health Care More Age-Friendly

Edited by
Judith L. Howe and Thomas V. Caprio

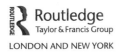
Routledge
Taylor & Francis Group

LONDON AND NEW YORK

First published 2020
by Routledge
2 Park Square, Milton Park, Abingdon, Oxon, OX14 4RN

and by Routledge
52 Vanderbilt Avenue, New York, NY 10017

Routledge is an imprint of the Taylor & Francis Group, an informa business

First issued in paperback 2021

Foreword, Chapters 1–4, 6–11 © 2020 Taylor & Francis
Chapter 5 is not subject to U.S. copyright law.

British Library Cataloguing-in-Publication Data
A catalogue record for this book is available from the British Library

ISBN13: 978-0-367-35288-2 (hbk)
ISBN13: 978-1-03-208978-2 (pbk)

Typeset in Minion Pro
by codeMantra

Publisher's Note
The publisher accepts responsibility for any inconsistencies that may have arisen during the conversion of this book from journal articles to book chapters, namely the inclusion of journal terminology.

Disclaimer
Every effort has been made to contact copyright holders for their permission to reprint material in this book. The publishers would be grateful to hear from any copyright holder who is not here acknowledged and will undertake to rectify any errors or omissions in future editions of this book.

Contents

CONTENTS

Citation Information

The chapters in this book were originally published in *Gerontology & Geriatrics Education*, volume 39, issue 2 (May 2018). When citing this material, please use the original page numbering for each article, as follows:

For any permission-related enquiries please visit:
http://www.tandfonline.com/page/help/permissions

Notes on Contributors

Ronald D. Adelman is the Medical Director of the Irving Wright Center of Aging and Co-Chief of the Division of Geriatrics Medicine and Gerontology at the New York-Presbyterian Hospital, USA. He is also a Professor of Clinical Medicine at Weill Cornell Medical College, New York City, USA.

Pam Ansell is the Director of Special Projects in the Division of Geriatrics and Gerontology at Weill Cornell Medical College, New York City, USA.

Julie Avanzino is a Program Representative at the University of California San Diego Center for Healthy Aging, USA.

Adrian G. Blundell is a Consultant Geriatrician and Honorary Associate Professor in Medicine of Older People in the Department of Health Care of Older People at Nottingham University Hospitals NHS Trust, UK.

Sara M. Bradley is an Associate Professor of Medicine in the Department of Medicine at Northwestern University Feinberg School of Medicine, Chicago, USA.

Mark Brennan-Ing is a Senior Research Scientist at Brookdale Center for Healthy Aging at Hunter College at the City University of New York, USA.

Jennifer Breznay is a Physician in the Division of Geriatrics at Maimonides Medical Center, USA.

Gwendolen T. Buhr is a Geriatric Medicine Specialist in the Division of Geriatrics at Duke University Medical Center, Durham, USA.

Kathryn E. Callahan is an Associate Professor of Gerontology and Geriatric Medicine in the Department of Internal Medicine in the Section on Hematology and Oncology at Wake Forest School of Medicine, Winston-Salem, USA.

Mary E. Camp is an Assistant Professor in the Department of Psychiatry at Southwestern Medical Center at the University of Texas, Dallas, USA.

Thomas V. Caprio is a Professor of Medicine, Geriatrics, Dentistry, Clinical Nursing, and Public Health Sciences at the University of Rochester Medical Center, USA.

Elizabeth Chapman is a Clinical Assistant Professor in Geriatrics in the Department of Medicine in the Geriatrics Division at the University of Wisconsin School of Medicine and Public Health, Madison, USA.

Colin A. Depp is a Professor in the Department of Psychiatry and the Director of Research Education and Training at the Clinical and Translational Research Institute at the University of California San Diego, USA, and a Clinical Psychologist in the VA San Diego Healthcare System, USA.

Alexis Eastman is a Physician and a Clinical Assistant Professor in the Department of Medicine in the Geriatrics Division at the University of Wisconsin School of Medicine and Public Health, Madison, USA.

James M. Fisher is a Consultant Geriatrician in Geriatric Medicine at Northumbria Healthcare NHS Foundation Trust, UK. He is also a Senior Lecturer at Newcastle University (Northumbria Base Unit), UK.

Mark J. Garside is a Specialist Registrar in Stroke and Elderly Care at Northumbria Healthcare NHS Foundation Trust, UK.

Maja Gawronska is the Public Relations and Events Manager at the University of California San Diego Center for Healthy Aging, USA.

Andrea Gilmore-Bykovskyi is an Assistant Professor at the University of Wisconsin School of Nursing, Madison, USA.

Adam L. Gordon is a Clinical Associate Professor in Medicine of Older People in the Division of Medical Sciences and Graduate Entry Medicine at the University of Nottingham, UK.

Debra Greenberg is an Instructor in the Department of Medicine in the Division of Geriatrics at Montefiore Medical Center, USA.

Mitchell Tod Heflin is a Professor of Medicine and a Senior Fellow in the Center for the Study of Aging and Human Development in the Department of Medicine at Duke University School of Medicine, Durham, USA.

Tina Hsu is an Assistant Professor of Medicine in the Division of Medical Oncology at Ottawa Hospital Cancer Centre, Canada.

Steven F. Huege is a Psychiatrist in the Department of Psychiatry at the University of California San Diego, USA.

Paul Jennings is a Mobile Intensive Care Ambulance Paramedic with Ambulance Victoria, Australia.

Haekyung Jeon-Slaughter is an Assistant Professor in the Department of Internal Medicine at Southwestern Medical Center at the University of Texas, Dallas, USA.

Dilip V. Jeste is the Senior Associate Dean for Healthy Aging and Senior Care at the University of California San Diego, USA.

Anne E. Johnson is an Assistant Professor in the Department of Psychiatry at Southwestern Medical Center at the University of Texas, Dallas, USA.

Victoria S. Kaprielian is the Associate Dean for Faculty Development and Medical Education at Campbell University School of Osteopathic Medicine, USA.

Reena Karani is a Professor and the Associate Dean for Undergraduate Medical Education and Curricular Affairs at the Icahn School of Medicine at Mount Sinai, New York City, USA.

Stephen E. Karpiak is the Associate Director of Research at ACRIA's Center on HIV and Aging, USA, and an Associate Faculty at New York University Rory Meyers College of Nursing, USA.

Amy Jo Kind is an Associate Professor of Geriatrics in the Department of Medicine in the Geriatrics Division in the School of Medicine and Public Health at the University of Wisconsin, Madison, USA, and an Attending Physician at the Geriatric Research Education and Clinical Center (GRECC) at William S Middleton Hospital in the United States Department of Veterans Affairs, USA.

Heidi D. Klepin is a Professor in the Department of Internal Medicine in the Section on Hematology and Oncology at Wake Forest School of Medicine, USA.

Beverly Lunsford is the Co-Director of the Center for Aging, Health and Humanities and an Assistant Professor at George Washington University School of Nursing, USA.

Ronald J. Maggiore is an Assistant Professor in the Department of Medicine in the Division of Hematology/Oncology at the University of Rochester, USA.

Catherine Nicastri is an Associate Professor in the Department of Medicine at Stony Brook School of Medicine, USA.

Colleen O'Connor Grochowski is the Associate Dean of Curricular Affairs at Duke University School of Medicine, Durham, USA.

Linda Pang is an Assistant Professor in the Department of General Internal Medicine at the University of Texas MD Anderson Cancer Center, Houston, USA.

Ira R. Parker is a Participant in the Cancer & Aging Research Group, USA.

Juliessa M. Pavon is a Geriatric Medicine Specialist in the Division of Geriatrics at Duke University Medical Center, Durham, USA.

Sandro O. Pinheiro is Associate Professor in Medicine and the Department of Community and Family Medicine, and Senior Fellow in the Center for Study of Aging at Duke University Medical Center, Durham, USA.

Laurie Posey is the Director of Nursing Education and an Associate Professor at George Washington University School of Nursing, USA.

Barrie L. Raik is a Physician in the Division of Geriatrics and Palliative Medicine at Weill Cornell Medical College, New York City, USA.

Tiffany Reed is a Physician at Piedmont Senior Care and Adult Medicine at Cone Health Medical Group, USA.

Linda Ross is a Senior Lecturer and the Deputy Head of the Department in the Department of Community Emergency Health & Paramedic Practice at Monash University, Australia.

John Z. Sadler is a Professor in the Department of Psychiatry at Southwestern Medical Center at the University of Texas, Dallas, USA.

Liz Seidel is the Clinical and Community Project Director for the Geriatric Workforce Enhancement Program at New York University Rory Meyers College of Nursing, USA.

Daniel D. Sewell is the Director of Senior Behavioral Health and a Professor in the Department of Psychiatry at the University of California San Diego, USA.

Janet A. Tooze is a Professor in the Department of Biostatistical Sciences at Wake Forest School of Medicine, USA.

Xin Tu is a Professor in Residence of Family Medicine and Public Health at the University of California San Diego, USA.

Bennett Vogelman is a Professor in the Department of Medicine at the University of Wisconsin School of Medicine and Public Health, Madison, USA.

Brett Williams is a Professor and the Head of the Department of Community Emergency Health and Paramedic Practice in the Faculty of Medicine, Nursing and Health Sciences at Monash University, Melbourne, Australia.

Mamata Yanamadala is an Assistant Professor of Medicine in the Department of Medicine at Duke University School of Medicine, Durham, USA.

Foreword

Clinical Education in Geriatrics: Innovative and Trusted Approaches Leading Workforce Transformation in Making Health Care More Age-Friendly

Thomas V. Caprio

In this issue of *Gerontology and Geriatrics Education* there is a focus on the ever-expanding activities in clinical education and training in geriatrics. In order to have the best prepared health care workforce, attention towards the unique needs of older adults has become a cornerstone of today's health professions curricula and continuing education. A strong emphasis in teaching has recently been placed on post-hospital discharge planning and navigating the complexities of transitions of care. This issue has three unique projects focusing on transitions. Linda Pang and colleagues worked with medical students in a reflective exercise on transitions to literally "bridge the gap" in assessing how patients cared for in the hospital made the journey to home. Pavon and colleagues developed a transitions of care curriculum for internal medicine interns covering the ACGME core competencies which can allow residency programs to hit the mark in multiple domains for learner assessment. Chapman and colleagues from Wisconsin immersed resident physicians in a real life peri-hospital experiential learning focused on transitions of care. These three trainings, while each unique, are especially important in helping participants understanding the role of the clinician as a stakeholder within the interprofessional team assisting older patients and their families navigating the complexities of the modern health system.

Ross and colleagues contribute an important systematic review of educational interventions aimed at improving student attitudes towards aging. Importantly this review underscores the powerful learning experiences of students obtained through the interactions with real patients. With such a focus in modern medical education on simulation, online training, and standardized patients for evaluation, it is important not to forget the end result of clinical training is to take care of real people. Mary Camp and colleagues contribute a poignant perspective on the patient interactions during training with analysis of the self-reflections in student essays related to geriatrics. The experiences with older adults during training, including moral distress experienced by students and the common challenges of aging encountered, likely contribute to the core professional identity development and attitudes of these students.

A framework of learning is explored by Yanamadala and colleagues in this issue through use of problem-based formats and by novel online "mini" e-learning modules to engage students as reported by Garside and colleagues. Beverly Lunsford and Laurie Posey outline a novel multimodal educational approach of "Geriatric education utilizing a palliative care framework" to enhance disease and symptom management and communication to provide compassionate care. A short-term research training program framework including didactic, clinical and methodology is described by Jeste and the team from the University of California. This program significantly and positively impacted medical students' attitudes toward aging. Programs which change perspectives in areas like research and palliative care may serve as powerful catalysts for creating a "pipeline" of students who embrace aging as a central theme of their work.

Geriatric fellowship training is also an important area for this issue. Mark Brennan-Ing and colleagues challenge the preconceptions that geriatric fellows may have regarding sexuality and sexual health in older age. In a powerful intervention directed towards geriatric fellows the team was able to alter perceptions about sexuality, health, and aging. Fellows were able to identify gaps in their own practices to better support older adults in sexual health. Finally, Ronald Maggiore and his colleagues in geriatric oncology also focused their work on geriatric fellows. A national survey of U.S. geriatrics fellowship program directors revealed strong support from programs in the principles of specialized cancer care for older adults but few have reported an operationalized geriatric oncology curriculum. This important identified gap creates ample opportunity for improving education especially when faced with the growing demographic imperative of an aging population with increasing prevalence of cancer.

It is a pleasure to have received such excellent submissions for this issue of *Gerontology and Geriatrics Education*. Health care workforce development is a critical issue in sensitizing clinicians to the needs of older adults. I would even propose instead of the term "development" we should refer to it as workforce "transformation" or "enhancement" with the goal to make health care more age-friendly. As demonstrated by these authors of articles related to clinical education, both innovation and trusted approaches in clinical teaching has the power to influence positive perspectives of students who will be at the forefront of this change in health care.

A problem-based learning curriculum in geriatrics for medical students

Mamata Yanamadala, Victoria S. Kaprielian, Colleen O'Connor Grochowski, Tiffany Reed, and Mitchell Tod Heflin

ABSTRACT

A geriatrics curriculum delivered to medical students was evaluated in this study. Students were instructed to review real patient cases, interview patients and caregivers, identify community resources to address problems, and present a final care plan. Authors evaluated the course feedback and final care plans submitted by students for evidence of learning in geriatric competencies. Students rated the efficacy of the course on a 5-point Likert scale as 3.70 for developing clinical reasoning skills and 3.69 for interdisciplinary teamwork skills. Assessment of an older adult with medical illness was rated as 3.87 and ability to perform mobility and functional assessment as 3.85. Reviews of written final care plans provided evidence of student learning across several different geriatric competencies such as falls, medication management, cognitive and behavior disorders, and self-care capacity. Assessment of the curriculum demonstrated that medical students achieved in-depth learning across multiple geriatric competencies through contact with real cases.

Introduction

The Institute of Medicine (IOM; 2008) has identified a critical need to expand geriatrics competence among all physicians. Older adults currently make up about 12% of the U.S. population, yet account for 26% of all physician office visits and 35% of all hospital stays. Effective care of this growing population requires knowledge and skills in the management of complex medical and psychosocial problems. In response, the IOM report recommends that all primary care and subspecialty physicians receive enhanced training in geriatrics. Unfortunately, deficiencies exist in preparation of medical students to care for geriatric patients in the United States. (Eleazer, Doshi, Wieland, Boland, & Hirth, 2005) As a result, students graduate with inadequate knowledge and skills in the care of older adults and, furthermore, may perceive geriatrics as a less valuable medical specialty and undesirable career option. (Anderson, 2004; Bagri & Tiberius, 2010; Ory, Kinney Hoffman, Hawkins, Sanner, & Mockenhaupt, 2003)

Color versions of one or more of the figures in the article can be found online at www.tandfonline.com/WGGE.

Over the last decade, grant-funded initiatives have targeted these deficiencies. Educators in geriatrics have applied novel strategies for medical student training, including senior mentor programs, community partnerships, and standardized patients. (Anderson, 2004) To provide consistent expectations for these efforts, a national taskforce published a set of minimum competencies in care of older adults for graduating medical students in 2009 (Leipzig et al., 2009). Significant efforts are underway to disseminate the competencies, but, to date, few models describing and evaluating experiences in medical schools to teach these competencies have been published (Atkinson, Lambros, & Davis et al., 2013).

Multiple barriers exist to effective instruction in geriatrics, including shortage of faculty and student time and funding. (Helms, Denson, Brown, & Simpson, 2009; Oates, Norton, & Russell et al., 2009; Strano-Paul, 2011; Sutin, Rolita, Yeboah, Taffel, & Zabar, 2011) Teaching geriatric competencies is also uniquely challenging for educators due to the complexity and multiplicity of medical, psychosocial, and functional issues. This complexity demands further development of effective and efficient curricula in geriatrics for medical students. Problem-based learning, particularly in examination of real cases, presents an educational strategy proven to enhance learning, particularly around psychosocial and teamwork issues so critical to geriatrics. (Koh, Khoo, Wong, & Koh, 2008) In this article we describe a week-long problem-based learning experience in geriatrics delivered to second-year medical students and its relative effectiveness in promoting learning geriatric competencies.

Method

Curriculum development

Interventions that include contact with older adults in a variety of settings have the highest success rates over time in increasing positive attitudes of medical students toward geriatric patients (Voogt, Mickus, Santiago, & Herman, 2008). In addition, problem-based learning (PBL) in medical school positively affects physician competencies essential to the care of older adults, including appreciation of social and ethical aspects of health care, communication skills, and self-directed learning. (Koh et al., 2008)

Review of the existing curriculum for medical students revealed opportunities to increase medical student interaction with geriatric patients. A subsequent curriculum revision led to the creation of a series of one-week intersessions between the standard clinical clerkships. These week-long experiences addressed key topics spanning multiple medical specialties, including geriatrics. Geriatrics faculty met regularly with the course director and administrators over a 6-month period to plan the curriculum. Given limited time, faculty elected to focus didactics and clinical experiences on selected core issues on care of older adults, including falls, cognitive impairment, polypharmacy, and caregiver stress.

Curriculum description

This week-long course titled "Clinical Core on Aging" was delivered to second-year medical students after completion of their first clinical clerkship. Learning objectives included the following:

By the end of the week, students will be able to:

(1) Analyze the case of an older adult suffering from one of four core problems (falls, polypharmacy, caregiver stress, or cognitive impairment) for root causes and contributing factors
(2) Cite evidence on the epidemiology of the problem, common contributing factors, and methods of prevention
(3) Describe community resources available to prevent or manage this core problem
(4) Propose specific recommendations at the patient and system level for improving care in this area
(5) Demonstrate teamwork skills.

We aimed to use a PBL strategy to teach teamwork, clinical reasoning, and care planning. PBL is defined as a method and philosophy, involving problem-first learning via work in small groups and independent study (Maudsley, 1999). This method encourages learners to use critical thinking and problem-solving skills as they apply content knowledge to real-world problems and issues.

During the week, students worked in teams of five on a project with a real patient affected by one or more of four core problems, including falls, cognitive decline, caregiver stress, and polypharmacy. Faculty reviewed and identified core issues for each case. Polypharmacy cases included not only those with multiple medications but also those with potentially inappropriate medications. Faculty and fellows recruited case patients by contacting primary providers in different settings including nursing homes, assisted living, independent living, community dwelling, and hospital. Course faculty aimed to achieve an even distribution of types of patient problems and locations of care among the student teams to optimize the value of discussions at the end of the week. Ten faculty members specializing in geriatrics and six geriatric fellows were recruited to conduct the introductory and final care plan discussions. In preparation for the week, faculty and fellows participated in an hour-long development session on PBL methodology.

The week-long course started with an introductory discussion of a real patient case (see Figure 1). This 90-minute small group discussion was facilitated by geriatric medicine faculty and fellow pairs. At the beginning of the session, students received a case packet that included a brief introductory paragraph describing the patient's age, gender, major medical problems, and chief concern or problem as well as resources and instructions for activities for the remainder of the week. With this information, students brainstormed a differential diagnosis for the brief information provided in the case. By the end of the session, student teams identified specific issues to research between sessions and a basic plan for their final presentation. On the afternoon of Day 1, students received a series of brief lectures on the core topics, including cognitive disorders, gait problems and falls, medication management, and caregiver stress. On Day 2, students performed an interview and assessment of the patient and (when possible) the caregiver. Students used Mini Mental Status Exam and Get Up and Go tools for cognitive and gait assessments, respectively (Folstein, Folstein, & McHugh, 1975; Podsiadlo & Richardson, 1991). In addition, they performed a systematic medication review that included dosage, timing, and indication of prescription and nonprescription drugs. They did not use a specific tool to assess caregiver burden. Interviews focused on the patient experience and the identification of causative factors for problems. Students were encouraged to begin to identify steps for prevention or management of subsequent events or problems. On Day 3 students met with members of the interdisciplinary team at a local continuing care retirement

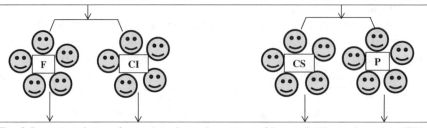

Figure 1. Organizational scheme for clinical core on aging.F = falls; CI = cognitive impairment; CS = caregiver stress; and P = polypharmacy.

community and then attended a panel discussion at the local senior center with representatives from Meals-on-Wheels, a nonprofit assisting older adults in managing medications, a publicly supported senior transportation agency, the State Health Insurance Information Program (SHIIP), caregiver support groups, and home care agencies. They also toured an Adult Day Health Program located there in the senior center.

Independent teamwork

Student teams also met independently in three predesignated 2-hour meeting times to work collaboratively on the patient case activity. Between meetings, students independently researched their patient's primary problem, etiology, and appropriate management strategies. Key references and contacts were provided for the core problems identified in their case. Faculty members were also available for questions during designated "office hours" for answering student questions.

Final activity

On the final day (Day 4), students met in large groups of four teams (20 students), each with a different core problem, to present their cases to each other. Teams took turns presenting with faculty facilitating the discussion. In their presentation, each team was directed to address the patient's problem(s), pertinent evidence from the literature, and approaches for the care of the patient. Although each case was linked with a core problem, they were allowed (and in some cases encouraged) to include discussion of other important problems. For example, if the core problem was dementia, but the patient had fallen, they could include this in the plan. At the end of the session, each student team comprising five students submitted a one-page paper summarizing their case, findings, and a plan of care. In the papers, they were asked to provide a brief synopsis of the case and then, based on their educational experiences and interactions over the course of the week, to identify specific problems and propose solutions.

Measures

Student self-assessment of learning

Students rated the efficacy of the course on a 5-point Likert-type scale (1 = *not at all successful*, 3 = *adequately successful*, 5 = *extremely successful*) on how successful the course was on achieving the following outcomes. The following evaluation items on the Likert-type scale were designed from the content taught in the course: (1) develop clinical reasoning skills, integrating knowledge to solve problems outside the confines of a single discipline; (2) develop skills and attitudes for effective interdisciplinary teamwork; (3) work with a team of providers to formulate a plan of care for an older adult with medical illness and functional decline; (4) perform assessments of mobility and function of an older adult; and (5) describe community resources to assist in management of common problems for older adults. Students were also asked to comment about the most effective aspect of the week, the most important thing they learned and provide suggestions for improvement.

Competency identification

As detailed above, students were asked to write a one-page paper on the case they investigated. The student papers were reviewed by two authors (MY and MTH) independently, looking for evidence of learning in the predefined minimum geriatrics-specific competencies addressed by the students (Leipzig et al., 2009). To qualify as "evidence of learning," the content of the papers needed to go beyond a simple mention of the problem to include all or most of the elements detailed in the competencies themselves. For example, if the students were allotted a case with falls as a core topic, they might have inquired about falls and performed a gait evaluation but did not provide an interpretation of the gait evaluation as required by the competency (One of the competency for the falls, gait, and balance reads as follows: Ask all patients > 65 years old, or their caregivers, about falls in the last year, watch the patient rise from a chair and walk (or transfer), and then record and interpret the findings).

We also identified relevant themes not necessarily listed among the competencies, such as financial issues or caregiver burden. No specific measures were defined to assess caregiver burden. Credit was given for student papers if they mentioned recognition of caregiver stress and strategies for management of caregiver stress. We used constant comparative analysis to review and reconcile findings over several rounds until consensus was achieved on themes identified in each paper. To evaluate the volume and frequency of competencies achieved, we calculated the median number of competencies addressed across teams and the percentage of teams that actually addressed the assigned core topic.

Institutional Review Board of our institution has exempted this research.

Results

Experience

Two hundred two students participated over two consecutive years in the program. There were 98 (48.5%) females and the group was ethnically diverse with 98 (48.5%) White students, 51 (25.2%) Asian, 42 (20.8%) African American, and 11 (5.4%) Hispanic. Students rated the efficacy of the course (1 = *not at all successful*, 5 = *extremely successful*) at 3.70 (*SD* = .89) for developing clinical reasoning skills and integrating knowledge to solve problems. Students rated their experience developing skills and attitudes for effective interdisciplinary teamwork as 3.69 (*SD* = .93). In terms of interdisciplinary team assessment of an older adult with medical illness and functional decline, students rated their experience as 3.87 (*SD* = .85). Efficacy in developing student ability to perform assessments of mobility and function of an older adult was rated as 3.85 (*SD* = .88). Efficacy in using community resources to assist in management of common problems for older adults was rated as 3.89 (*SD* = .95).

Student comments reflected general acceptance of PBL methods: "The team-based activity was extremely engaging and practical—actually working with real patients was tremendously effective relative to standard classroom based learning" and

> I thought it was working with actual patients and making suggestions to improve their care was the best part [sic]. Health care team visits with real patients better highlighted the complexities and intricacies of aging and chronic disease better than any lecture or textbook.

Evidence of learning for competencies: Which competencies were addressed?

Review of 40 final papers revealed that student teams addressed competencies across at total of seven different domains (Figure 2). The average number of total competencies addressed in each paper were 2.5, and the average number of additional geriatric pertinent issues (identified but not listed in the competencies) were 1.44 per each paper. Sixty-three percent of student papers addressed at least one to two competencies, whereas 24% papers addressed three to four

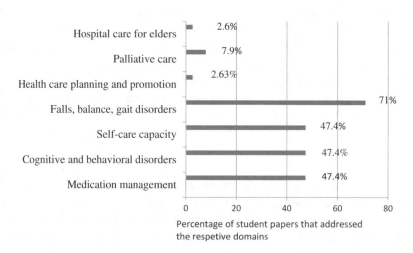

Figure 2. Frequency of geriatric competencies addressed by domain in final papers.

competencies, and 10% addressed five to six competencies. Students most commonly described issues with falls, balance, and gait (71%). Medication management, cognitive and behavior disorders, and self-care capacity were addressed in 47.4% of the papers (Figure 2). In addition to the predefined competencies the content in students' papers reflected learning in key geriatric content areas including caregiver challenges in 47.4% and pain assessment and management in 23.7%. Learners evaluated financial issues, identified community resources for the elderly and discussed advance directives in about 15% of the papers (Figure 3). Below are two examples from student papers that included final care plans and system changes to impact outcomes for older patients.

(1) In a case of 93-year-old male rehospitalized after recent hospitalization due to poor transitions in care, the student team suggested "empowering elderly patients to take more active role during the transition by educating patient and caregiver about care plan and the elderly playing an active role in devising their post discharge plan. Keeping up with current medication list by informing all parties about changes. Care settings operating as silos can be detrimental to patients and propose communication of care plans between settings."

(2) Another case was of 83-year-old female with dementia living independently at home with her husband was requiring assistance with activities of daily living and the husband is experiencing care giving burden and would like to continue to stay at home. The husband was feeling isolated due to lack of social interaction. The team suggested "attending free congregate lunch program offered by the local Center for senior life to increase social interaction and suggestions for free respite care and care giver support program and involvement with a book club in library to encourage his favorite activity."

How often did they explicitly address their assigned core topic?

Interestingly, students did not always clearly address their assigned "core" issue (Table 1). Ninety percent of those assigned to address caregiver issues did so, as did 87% of those assigned to a case with falls as the core topic. However, only 72% of those assigned to a

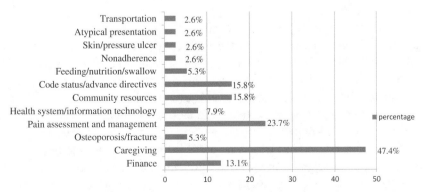

Percentage of student papers that addressed additional geriatric content areas

Figure 3. Frequency of identification of other geriatric issues in final papers.

Table 1. Competencies Addressed in Student Final Papers.

	Cognitive Impairment ($n = 11$)	Polypharmacy ($n = 8$)	Fall ($n = 8$)	Caregiver stress ($n = 11$)
Competency addressed in student papers for the core problem of the case (%)	72	62	87	90.9
Additional competencies addressed in student papers (average)	1.27	0.87	1.5	2
Additional geriatric content areas addressed (average)	1.18	1.375	0.87	1

dementia case, and 62% of those with medication management successfully addressed these issues. When students did not address the core issue it was because they did not achieve the level of discussion necessary to count as evidence of learning. In some cases students addressed issues other than the assigned core issues.

Discussion

Assessment of the week-long PBL activity through course evaluation and review of the final papers demonstrated that medical students achieved in-depth learning across multiple geriatric competencies through contact with real cases in a PBL format. Given involvement of caregivers in the interview process this became a natural focus of the student papers. Likewise, falls are an important focal event for older adults and their caregivers and were frequently addressed in student papers. Medications and dementia were not as frequently addressed by the students. This underperformance in the domains of dementia and polypharmacy was seen in both years and certainly suggests a need for a greater emphasis in the curriculum in these areas in the future. In addition, identification and management of medication problems and cognitive impairment require deliberate and systematic approaches that these novice students may lack. Further clarification of student performance expectations may help address problems with learner performance. Although the student teams were instructed to focus on one core geriatric problem, the qualitative review of their final papers showed that they were able to identify and address other domains in the minimum geriatric competencies as well. Students also recognized and researched other common geriatric issues in the management of geriatric patients that were not included in the competencies, such as financial issues, pain assessment and management, advance directives, and others.

The clinical core in aging experience allowed for richer learning as the students interacted with real patients and connected with community resources. Interaction with real people added value to student interactions and lent a broader perspective about their patients that could not have been achieved with didactics alone or simulated cases. In person interaction with interprofessional health care providers and community resources permitted the learners to have interactive discussions that enhanced their learning.

Implementing the week-long PBL activity was logistically complex in terms of selecting cases with a variety of pertinent problems from a variety of settings, and assigning them to teams. This also involved scheduling a significant number of preceptors for the events. Alternative teaching methods instead of real cases, such as classroom-based activities or simulation used in other studies, might have been less complex logistically and more easily sustainable. One study focused on integration of competencies through e-learning. (Helms et al., 2009) Another study had a month-long multisite fourth-year geriatrics clerkship using an ambulatory and home care geriatrics program (Oates et al., 2009) while two other studies used Observed Structured Clinical Examinations to supplement the teaching and assessment of geriatrics skills (Strano-Paul, 2011; Sutin et al., 2011). These models successfully introduced students to several geriatrics competencies, but these curricula required longer periods of time and were sometimes personnel intensive. Such programs may be difficult to implement in many institutions with limited geriatrics resources and different curricular structures. One other model was a week-long curriculum that was successful in introducing the geriatric competencies. (Atkinson et al., 2013) This one-week model included primarily clinical encounters with patients in the hospital, clinic, long-term care, and independent living in addition to reading assignments. This program along with our model demonstrates that the competencies could be addressed in a short period of time with or without geriatric specific settings.

The PBL approach used in this activity encouraged learners to use critical-thinking and problem-solving skills as they applied content knowledge to real case problems. Group-based activities and interaction with interdisciplinary personnel helped learners appreciate social aspects of caring for older adults. Literature suggests that PBL in medical school positively affects physician competencies essential to the care of older adults, including appreciation of social and ethical aspects of health care, communication skills, and lifelong learning. (Koh et al., 2008) The outcomes from this activity demonstrated similar outcomes seen in literature from PBL activities.

This study has a few important limitations. To avoid survey burden, we did not perform a formal measure of students' attitudes. Evaluation measures were limited to those performed at week's end. More distal measures may have demonstrated how students retained and even applied concepts learned. In the future, this type of curriculum would lend itself to use summative measures at the end of clinical training such as observed structured clinical exam (OSCE) or clinical evaluation exercise (CEX).

Improvements noted in clinical reasoning skills and recognition of importance of interdisciplinary teamwork were based on students' self-evaluations. More objective measures of these constructs, a pretest, and a comparison group would be needed to make stronger conclusions about the effectiveness of the PBL in these domains.

This PBL activity demonstrated knowledge application to real cases. Follow-up evaluation to determine the effectiveness of this activity in future practice will be a next step for studying the effect on practice change. The impact of student recommendations on actual cases in solving real problems for the patients could also be evaluated.

Conclusions

Introduction of a PBL exercise provided an effective means of educating second-year medical students on core geriatrics subjects, while helping students to develop clinical reasoning skills, recognize importance of interdisciplinary teamwork, and understand key social and ethical issues in geriatrics on self-evaluations. Future steps should include more objective measurements to determine the effectiveness of the PBL in these domains.

Acknowledgments

This curriculum is made possible with help from geriatrics faculty and geriatric fellows at the Division of Geriatrics, Duke University.

Funding

The authors would like to thank the following for funding this research: Donald W. Reynolds Program for Faculty Development to Advance Geriatrics Education, Health Resources and Services Administration Geriatric Training for Physicians, Dentists and Mental Health Professionals Grant (D01HP08791), Geriatric Academic teaching award, Duke School of Medicine.

References

Anderson, M. B. (2004). A thematic summary of the geriatrics curricula at 40 US medical schools. *Academic Medicine*, *79*(7), S213–S222. doi:10.1097/00001888-200407001-00044

Atkinson, H. H., Lambros, A., Davis, B. R., Lawlor, J.S., Lovato, J., Sink, K.M., … Williamson, J.D. (2013). Teaching medical student geriatrics competencies in 1 week: An efficient model to teach and document selected competencies using clinical and community resources. *Journal of the American Geriatrics Society*, *61*, 1182–1187. doi:10.1111/jgs.12314

Bagri, A. S., & Tiberius, R. (2010). Medical student perspectives on geriatrics and geriatric education. *Journal of the American Geriatrics Society*, *58*(10), 1994–1999. doi:10.1111/j.1532-5415.2010.03074.x

Eleazer, G. P., Doshi, R., Wieland, D., Boland, R., & Hirth, V. A. (2005). Geriatric content in medical school curricula: Results of a national survey. *Journal of the American Geriatrics Society*, *53*(1), 136–140. doi:10.1111/jgs.2005.53.issue-1

Folstein, M.F., Folstein, S.E., McHugh, P.R. (1975). "Mini-mental state." A practical method for grading the cognitive state of patients for the clinician. *Journal of Psychiatric Research*, *12*(3), 189–198.

Helms, A., Denson, K., Brown, D., & Simpson, D. (2009). One specialty at a time: Achieving competency in geriatrics through an e-learning neurology clerkship module. *Academic Medicine*, *84*(10), S67–S69. doi:10.1097/ACM.0b013e3181b37a38

Institute of Medicine. (2008). *Retooling for an aging America: building the health care workforce*. Washington, DC: National Academies Press.

Koh, G. C.-H., Khoo, H. E., Wong, M. L., & Koh, D. (2008). The effects of problem-based learning during medical school on physician competency: A systematic review. *Canadian Medical Association Journal*, *178*(1), 34–41. doi:10.1503/cmaj.070565

Leipzig, R. M., Granville, L., Simpson, D., Anderson, M. B., Sauvigné, K., & Soriano, R. P. (2009). Keeping Granny safe on July 1: A consensus on minimum geriatrics competencies for graduating medical students. *Academic Medicine*, *84*(5), 604–610. doi:10.1097/ACM.0b013e31819fab70

Maudsley, G. (1999). Do we all mean the same thing by "problem-based learning"? A review of the concepts and a formulation of the ground rules. *Academic Medicine: Journal of the Association of American Medical Colleges*, *74*(2), 178–185. doi:10.1097/00001888-199902000-00016

Oates, D. J., Norton, L. E., Russell, M. L., Chao, S.H., Hardt, E.J., Brett, B., … Levine, S.A. (2009). Multisite geriatrics clerkship for fourth-year medical students: A successful model for teaching the Association of American Medical Colleges' Core Competencies. *Journal of the American Geriatrics Society*, *57*(10), 1917–1924. doi:10.1111/j.1532-5415.2009.02449.x

Ory, M., Kinney Hoffman, M., Hawkins, M., Sanner, B., & Mockenhaupt, R. (2003). Challenging aging stereotypes: Strategies for creating a more active society. *American Journal of Preventive Medicine*, *25*(3), 164–171. doi:10.1016/S0749-3797(03)00181-8

Podsiadlo, D., Richardson, S. (1991). "Up & Go" A test of basic functional mobility for frail elderly persons. *Journal of American Geriatrics Society*. *39*(2), 142–148.

Strano-Paul, L. (2011). Effective teaching methods for geriatric competencies. *Gerontology & Geriatrics Education*, *32*(4), 342–349. doi:10.1080/02701960.2011.611557

Sutin, D., Rolita, L., Yeboah, N., Taffel, L., & Zabar, S. (2011). A novel longitudinal geriatric medical student experience: Using teaching objective structured clinical examinations. *Journal of the American Geriatrics Society*, *59*(9), 1739–1744. doi:10.1111/j.1532-5415.2011.03538.x

Voogt, S. J., Mickus, M., Santiago, O., & Herman, S. E. (2008). Attitudes, experiences, and interest in geriatrics of first-year allopathic and osteopathic medical students. *Journal of the American Geriatrics Society*, *56*(2), 339–344. doi:10.1111/(ISSN)1532-5415

The development and evaluation of mini-GEMs – short, focused, online e-learning videos in geriatric medicine

Mark J. Garside, James M. Fisher, Adrian G. Blundell, and Adam L. Gordon

ABSTRACT

Mini Geriatric E-Learning Modules (Mini-GEMs) are short, focused, e-learning videos on geriatric medicine topics, hosted on YouTube, which are targeted at junior doctors working with older people. This study aimed to explore how these resources are accessed and used. The authors analyzed the viewing data from 22 videos published over the first 18 months of the Mini-GEM project. We conducted a focus group of U.K. junior doctors considering their experiences with Mini-GEMS. The Mini-GEMs were viewed 10,291 times over 18 months, equating to 38,435 minutes of total viewing time. The average viewing time for each video was 3.85 minutes. Learners valued the brevity and focused nature of the Mini-GEMs and reported that they watched them in a variety of settings to supplement clinical experiences and consolidate learning. Watching the videos led to an increase in self-reported confidence in managing older patients. Mini-GEMs can effectively disseminate clinical teaching material to a wide audience. The videos are valued by junior doctors due to their accessibility and ease of use.

Introduction

The world's population is aging—by 2050 two billion people will be age older than age 60 years (United Nations, 2015). Doctors must receive specific training to meet the health care needs of this group. National survey data from the United Kingdom in 2013 found the median time devoted to formal teaching about geriatric medicine was only 55 hours out of a 5-year program (Gordon et al., 2014). Harnessing innovative teaching methods, such as technology-enhanced learning (TEL), may help to address this training deficit (Oakley et al., 2014).

TEL is increasingly used and accepted in geriatric medicine. Computer-aided learning (CAL) in core geriatric medicine topics, used as part of a blended learning approach, has been associated with improved student examination performance (Daunt et al., 2013). The Portal of Geriatrics Online Education (POGOe) provides access to an array of TEL resources (Ramaswamy et al., 2015). Emerging technologies such as these represent a

Color versions of one or more of the figures in the article can be found online at www.tandfonline.com/WGGE.

paradigm shift in medical education. Among medical educators there is increasing support for this concept of high-quality, free, open-access "Meducation" (FOAM)(Shaw, 2013).

The application of social media, such as YouTube and Twitter (Forgie, Duff, & Ross, 2013), is increasingly being used in delivery of medical education (Nolan, 2011). Mobile learning, using Internet-enabled devices, has potential to improve the reach of medical education due to widespread device ownership (Nolan, 2011) coupled with a willingness to use technology to access content (Ellaway, Fink, Graves, & Campbell, 2014). It is crucial that clinical teachers who use these technologies are creative and critical in their implementation. Considering "pedagogy before technology'" emphasizes rational application of technologies within proven practices and models of teaching (Beetham & Sharpe, 2007).

Against this background we developed novel geriatric medicine teaching resources optimized for mobile learning, distributed via social media and designed to be brief. Mini Geriatric E-Learning Modules (Mini-GEMs) are short, focused, online video slide-shows aimed at junior doctors who care for older people. We describe here their development and evaluation.

Method

Development of mini-GEMs

Aim

Mini-GEMs were developed to provide an geriatric medicine–specific educational resource that followed the principles of FOAM. The intention was to build a library of topics with key learning points that could be accessed easily and quickly by busy clinical learners. The primary target audience was junior doctors, but the materials were created with the intention that they could be of interest to a wide range of clinical staff who work with older patients.

Style

PechaKucha (Japanese for "chit-chat") is a presentation format, developed in the early 2000s, that specifies speakers use 20 slides, for 20 seconds each (Beyer, 2011). We hypothesized that this format would fit well with mobile opportunistic learning .

Theoretical considerations informing design

The predominant learning theories that informed the design of the Mini-GEMs were cognitive load (Lau, 2014) and multimedia design theories. These consider processing of audio, visual, and textual information (Sandars, Patel, Goh, Kokatailo, & Lafferty, 2015) and describe the capacity of working memory to be limited, with learning becoming more difficult if the cognitive load of a task exceeds this limit (Young, Van Merrienboer, Durning, & Ten Cate, 2014). Mini-GEMs were designed to minimize cognitive load by restricting information on each slide, ensuring slide layout was minimalist and providing time for learners to attend to content.

Target audience

Mini-GEMs were designed for junior doctors. Each Mini-GEM is designed to cover a specific topic relevant to clinical practice (the Mini-GEMs library is available to view at aeme.org.uk/mini-gems).

Software and host platform

We chose to host the Mini-GEMs on YouTube, based on its popularity and broad compatibility with Internet-connected devices, No login is required, and there are few bandwidth issues with modern devices in developed countries.

Authors & process

Mini-GEM authors were initially drawn from the Association of Elderly Medicine Education (AEME)—a nonprofit organization seeking to advance education of health care professionals caring for older patients. Initial topics were selected among the group, based on clinical interests of authors. Once the format had been launched, and the library of videos began to grow, AEME were contacted by geriatricians throughout the United Kingdom who were keen to create their own Mini-GEM. Topics were jointly agreed between authors and the AEME committee, to ensure a breadth of content that would be clinically relevant to junior medical staff working with older patients. The electronic nature of the material made remote recording of content feasible. The process of creating a Mini-GEM is summarized below:

(1) Authors design their slideshow presentation on their own computer, following standardized formatting guidelines provided.
(2) The slides are internally peer reviewed by two "editors" at AEME to ensure clarity and accuracy—following any required revisions, the presentation is agreed with the author.
(3) The author records narration for each slide using either voice recording software on their smartphone or a computer microphone.
(4) The slides and audio are reformatted centrally to ensure uniformity of style and are then combined to form a video slideshow which is uploaded to YouTube.

Evaluation of mini-GEMs

Mini-GEMs were evaluated using a synthesis of objective and participant-orientated evaluation (Cook, 2010). We were not seeking to demonstrate that watching Mini-GEMs improved objective knowledge, but rather to describe if, how, and why this format of educational resource would be utilized by clinicians.

The aim of the objectives-orientated evaluation was to determine the uptake of Mini-GEMs and viewer characteristics. Data was collected using YouTube's built-in analytic software that provided information on the number and duration of views, geographical location of viewers, and devices used.

The aim of the participant-orientated evaluation was to explore how users engaged with Mini-GEMs, and their attitudes toward the resources having done so. This was done using a focus group. Participants were attendees at "Geriatrics for Juniors"—a U.K. national conference for junior doctors interested in geriatric medicine. Delegates were sent invites before the conference asking them to join the focus group if they had used Mini-GEMs. Participants were selected on a first-come, first served basis. The focus group was chaired by AG, a consultant geriatrician independent of the Mini-GEM project. The discussion followed a semistructured topic guide (see the appendix), which was generated to explore how, why, and when users accessed the Mini-GEMs and to describe their experiences of, and attitudes toward, them. The topic guide was allowed to develop freely during the focus group as areas of interest arose. Discussions were digitally recorded and manually transcribed.

Thematic analysis followed an interpretative phenomenological approach (Bunniss & Kelly, 2010), as we were looking to explore and describe participants' experience of, and interaction with, the educational material. Transcripts were initially reviewed and coded independently by two researchers (MG, JF), with the aim of identifying patterns and themes in the data. The researchers then met to discuss the coding frameworks produced. Consensus was reached by merging similar codes and iterative joint review of the data until a final thematic structure was agreed (Figure 2). Potentially contradictory evidence was sought and considered against emergent themes (negative case analysis), a process recognized as being critical to rigorous analysis (Barbour, 2001).

Ethics

Ethical approval was not required for this study, as participants were all either employed by or affiliated with the NHS. This was confirmed by the local Research Ethics Committee. All participants signed a consent form prior to the focus group, outlining how the data would be gathered, stored, and used.

Results

YouTube analytics

YouTube analytics were downloaded 18 months after the initial Mini-GEM was published. These showed 22 videos published by 15 authors with a combined total of 10,291 views, and 38,435 minutes of viewing time. Content was accessed from 110 countries (76% United Kingdom). An example of audience retention data from YouTube analytics is shown in Figure 1. This is typical of audience retention patterns seen across the Mini-GEMs library with significant audience loss within the first 20 seconds, followed by a more gradual loss thereafter. Only 30% of initial viewers were still watching at the video's end.

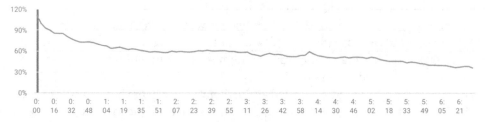

Figure 1. An example audience retention graph provided by YouTube analytics, showing the number of views for every moment of a video as a percentage of the total number of video views.

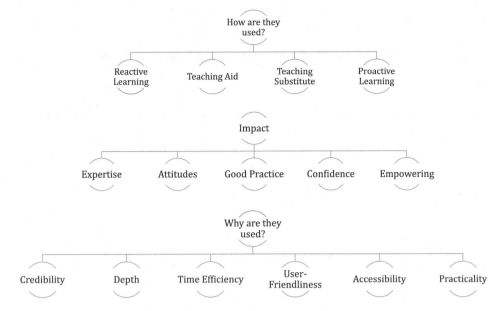

Figure 2. Thematic coding framework.

The average viewing duration was 3 minutes and 44 seconds, equating to 54% of the available video. Full viewing and retention data for all the Mini-GEMs is shown in Table 1.

Focus-group data

The focus group consisted of six junior doctors, with between 1 and 4 years postgraduate experience, and one final year medical student, from across the United Kingdom.

Thematic analysis of transcripts identified three main themes, with no significant disagreements between the researchers:

- Why learners had chosen to use Mini-GEMs
- How Mini-GEMs were incorporated into existing learning frameworks
- The perceived impact of Mini-GEMs on clinical work.

Why use mini-GEMs?

Participants identified that Mini-GEMs were easily accessible on mobile devices and contrasted this with previous experiences of TEL:

> The ease of accessing them ... for someone who's gone to different hospitals who has had to do online modules ... it was an absolute pleasure to literally press it, it was on YouTube, I had it on my iPad, it was so simple, rather than putting in fifteen million passwords ... I pressed play once and it worked (Participant #2).

The short duration of the Mini-GEMs was attractive to junior doctors and enabled them to undertake ad-hoc learning not practicable with lengthier resources, "I know that I have five minutes free with a quick cup of tea and that I can play it. But that if it's an hour it's more daunting and I'm like 'do I have time to do that'?" (Participant #6) and "I think the thing about

Table 1. Viewing and Retention Data for Mini-GEMs (from July 11, 2013 to July, 5, 2015).

Topic	Date Uploaded	Video Length (Minutes)	Total Hours Watched	Views	Average View Duration (Minutes)	Average % of Content Viewed	% Viewers Watching at the End
Introduction to Mini-GEMs	07/11/13	6.02	16.90	400	2.53	42	25
Stroke Thrombolysis	12/12/13	6.02	56.40	1100	3.08	51	22
Parkinson's Disease	09/01/14	6.32	18.95	353	3.22	51	31
Delirium	06/02/14	6.98	62.85	1013	3.72	53	34
Assessment Following a Fall	12/03/14	7.37	41.85	553	4.54	61	36
Polypharmacy	13/03/14	7.40	65.75	978	4.03	54	34
Dementia	17/03/14	5.77	17.58	353	2.99	51	36
Urinary Tract Infections (UTIs)	09/04/14	6.35	60.92	901	4.06	63	40
Constipation	13/05/14	7.47	29.85	390	4.59	61	35
"Acopia"	25/06/14	6.88	27.02	409	3.96	57	38
Tips for New Docs	23/07/14	7.12	19.02	274	4.17	58	34
Palliative Care	11/08/14	6.62	11.88	173	4.12	62	44
Mental Capacity	13/08/14	6.62	114.78	1955	3.52	53	36
Dizziness	01/10/14	7.98	30.25	414	4.39	54	33
Atypical Presentations	26/10/14	6.95	17.80	281	3.80	54	38
Do Not Attempt Cardio-pulmonary Resuscitation (DNACPR) Decisions	30/12/14	7.95	16.78	205	4.91	61	46
Fluids	19/01/15	7.43	6.93	102	4.08	54	29
Urinary Incontinence	05/03/15	5.27	6.18	120	3.09	58	31
Surgical Diagnoses	13/03/15	8.00	6.78	110	3.70	46	28
The Geriatrician's Profanisaurus	11/04/15	5.17	7.23	133	3.26	63	52
The Epley Manoeuvre	13/04/15	5.57	3.88	59	3.95	71	44
Myeloma	15/03/15	6.78	0.92	11	5.03	74	NA[a]
Average (Mean)		6.73	29.12	468	3.85	57	36

Note. UTIs = ; DNACPR =
a. Not enough views to generate audience retention data.

them being short is that it is not daunting to go and sit down when you've come in from a long day at work and you're tired" (Participant #3).

The reliable nature of the format, where viewers were aware of the prespecified duration of the content, was also appealing, since the "risk" of wasted time was minimized:

> You can get drawn into thinking something might be useful and then realising it's not quite what you're looking for. Whereas these are positive in two ways—they're short enough so that you could watch the whole five minutes, and even if you thought that wasn't useful it's only five minutes (Participant #7).

Mini-GEMs focused on commonly encountered scenarios for health care professionals caring for older people—viewers spoke about the clinical relevance of the content, which they felt helped facilitate translation of acquired knowledge into practice:

> Because they relate to patients you see all the time it seems more likely that it'll stick in your head (Participant #1).
> What I really like about them most is that they teach you how to approach patients. So they give you an apparatus, a system, an attitude or a structure to take with you, so that when you do go and see these patients … you (are) in the right frame of mind (Participant #5).

Participants highlighted that Mini-GEMs did not provide an exhaustive overview. Although further work was required to learn in-depth about a subject, participants spoke about this in positive terms:

> It's a short, concise version of something that's giving you concepts rather than firm details of it. So if you find something where you think hang on, I'm not quite sure I know the details of that, you know you can go and look it up (Participant #3).

How are mini-GEMs being used?

Participants described various contexts where they used the videos. These included prior to geriatric medicine attachments, to complement revision for postgraduate examinations, to aid reflection following clinical experiences, and as an aide memoir prior to seeing an older patient:

> I knew what the topics were, and then I got asked to see someone on the ward with a fall. So I thought "OK, because [there's] not that much of a rush, I've got five minutes or whatever I'll watch it first to give myself a bit of a refresher" (Participant #1).

Participants suggested that the Mini-GEMs felt similar to ward-based clinical teaching delivered by peers or senior colleagues, "It wasn't in a patronising way, it was in a comforting way, almost like you were being taught by one of your registrars" (Participant #2).

Participants seemed to attach credibility to Mini-GEMs because the focus of the teaching was similar to informal ward-based teaching by senior colleagues but also because senior colleagues within the specialty could be trusted to know what they were talking about, "What gives these credibility? (AG)

> I guess because they're … done by registrars and consultants working in the specialty (Participant #1).
> And why do you assume that they know what they are talking about? (AG)
> You have to trust seniors to teach and it just kind of comes down (to that) (Participant #1).

What is the impact of mini-GEMs on clinical practice?

Participants reported that Mini-GEMs increased their confidence in dealing with clinical problems:

> [The Mini-GEMs have] given me more confidence in what I previously thought. I wouldn't say there was anything ground-breaking on the ones that I looked at but they made me feel a bit more happy, can I say, with what I was already doing (Participant #2).

Mini-GEMs helped reinforce good clinical practice and in some cases participants felt empowered to act more autonomously than they had done previously:

> I think a lot of people are, you know, dealing with patients on their own most of the time and yes, you have access to a senior or a registrar, but you know, you want to make sure that you're doing something for them yourself (Participant #5).

In addition to clinical knowledge and skills, there was a suggestion that Mini-GEMs might inspire viewers to challenge suboptimal attitudes and approaches to the care of older patients:

> I would love to play them to some consultants that you're on take with and just think actually, the three minutes you just spent with that patient is not an adequate amount of time... "Oh, it's just a UTI" or "Oh it's a fall," kind of simplifying things that are common in the elderly but beneath them have a whole multitude of causes (Participant #7).

Participants reported a willingness to promote and share the resources among junior colleagues and medical students, including those working outside the field of geriatric medicine, "I talked to my housemate about them, she is interested in General Practice— there are some similarities ... she was quite interested that there were these snippets online" (Participant #6) and "I think they'd be useful to show ... to some of my colleagues in surgery who feel medically unsupported ... as a sort of succinct survival guide" (Participant #7).

Disadvantages of mini-GEMs?

> We revisited the transcripts several times looking for accounts of negative aspects, or limitations of the Mini-GEMs. Although it was clear that the facilitator sought to elicit these, there were no comments from participants that suggested dissatisfaction with the Mini-GEMs, nor any suggestions for how they could be improved.

Discussion

This study describes the theoretical framework underpinning the development of the Mini-GEMs and an evaluation using robust measures of use and usability. A separate qualitative evaluation helped develop a more detailed understanding of how and why users accessed Mini-GEMs and how they benefitted from doing so. The main findings are:

- Mini-GEMs have been widely accessed, in terms of numbers and geographic distribution of viewership
- An average of 36% of all viewers followed the Mini-GEMs through to their end
- Junior doctors valued them because of accessibility, brevity, simplicity and the credibility of presenters and the material presented.

The Mini-GEMs were viewed on mobile devices and shared and accessed via social media. The consistent style and format created a sense of brand familiarity among users, enabling them to plan how to incorporate them into their learning. Hosting concise content on a readily accessible forum increased convenience for the learners.

It has been argued elsewhere that promoting accessibility of concise, digestible content may lead to "superficial learning," with failure to internalize knowledge and that this might render learners reliant on revisiting the content (Wallace, Clark, & White, 2012). Against this, though viewers acknowledged that the brevity of Mini-GEMs limited the amount of content that could be addressed, they reported that they used the mini-GEMs as a supplement to, rather than replacement for, other educational resources, thus allowing depth learning through reinforcement.

The Mini-GEMs were used in a variety of ways. They were used to facilitate knowledge acquisition during exam revision, before starting elderly care placements and for consolidation after clinical encounters. Mini-GEMs also provided learners with frameworks and schemata for the evaluation of an older patient they recognised as generalizable to broader practice.

Mini-GEMs may have influenced learners' attitudes towards older people. One participant described a desire to challenge suboptimal attitudes to care of older people with frailty. Her comments suggested higher-level reflection on the learning and the development of insight that practice could be improved. Negative attitudes about older patients have been recognized, even within doctors who have expressed an interest in geriatric medicine (Fisher, Hunt, & Garside, 2014)—more work is needed to explore educational strategies that address these attitudes.

Mini-GEMs were used "on the job," enabling "reactive learning"—that is unplanned but intentional learning that "takes place almost spontaneously in response to recent, current or imminent situations" (Eraut, 2000). The use of learning videos as refreshers in the workplace is established for procedure-based content (Topps, Helmer, & Ellaway, 2013), but we had not anticipated that geriatric medicine resources, which are less protocol driven, would be used in this manner. This demonstrates the potential for TEL to supplant or compliment the more traditional quick-reference textbooks frequently used.

Watching a Mini-GEM maybe considered passive learning due to lack of user interaction with the video. It has been suggested that medical students may prefer passive learning experiences when fatigued (Yavner et al., 2015). To strengthen the sociocollaborative element of learning, Twitter-based discussion related to the content of newly uploaded Mini-GEMs has been encouraged. Combining the Mini-GEMs with other learning resources may produce more effective learning—for example, the "flipped classroom" approach may be a potential way to integrate TEL and face-to-face learning (Moffett, 2015).

Analyzing audience retention data enabled us to understand users' viewing habits. The initial loss of viewers is likely to represent viewers who rapidly realized that they had no interest in the subject matter, or who had mistakenly accessed the content. However, the more gradual decline in cumulative viewing time over the length of each video suggests that even for those viewers who continue watching beyond the initial introduction, interest was lost over time. Further work is required to determine the optimum duration for this style of educational resource.

There is potential for resources such as the Mini-GEMs to be used to support clinical education in the care of older adults outside the specialty of geriatric medicine, which may be an important aspect of improving standards of care for all older patients within the health care system.

Limitations

Caution is needed when interpreting data derived from YouTube's proprietary software—there are challenges associated with overinterpreting multiple variables gleaned from a relatively small cohort. In addition, the true meaning of some of these variables must be caveated. A "view," for example, may not have actually constituted a true viewing. We have no record of what the learner was doing or thinking at that time (Ellaway, 2013).

Similarly, the demographics of individual viewers is unknown—It is not possible to determine whether the viewers were clinicians or interested members of the public, thus making interpretation of viewer retention statistics challenging. Insisting learners register to enable content to be accessed may facilitate profiling of users, but doing so would add a barrier to access that may deter some users and is contrary to the principles of FOAM (Shaw, 2013). The ease with which viewers could access the videos was one of the key strengths of the format highlighted by the focus group.

Our focus group participants were all United Kingdom based and were recruited at a conference on geriatric medicine. As delegates at such a conference, they may already have an innate enthusiasm for the specialty, and their views may not be representative of the broader community of clinicians accessing the Mini-GEMs, who may have different international perspectives and may be approaching the material with less enthusiasm for the specialty.

We acknowledge that this evaluation does not provide evidence of knowledge acquisition. This was by design, because meta-analysis level evidence already exists demonstrating that online e-learning is associated with significant knowledge gains (Cook et al., 2008). Instead, the aim was to evaluate perceived strengths and weaknesses of the format in the "real world" (i.e., *why* it works) and to explore utilization of the resource (i.e., how it works). Cook et al. (2008) described how such research questions (forming so-called clarification studies), are rarely considered and how it is crucial that they are addressed if the science of medical education research is to be advanced.

It is important to recognize that insights generated from YouTube analytics and a single focus group will be limited in terms of generalizability to a wider audience. However, these represent more detailed evaluations than commonly presented in articles sharing innovative e-learning packages (Eskildsen, 2010). They deliver some important insights into the putative impact of the Mini-GEMs and suggest some possible areas for future investigation and project development. Ideally, the thematic framework that has emerged from the work undertaken so far should be further explored through more focus groups, and questionnaire surveys attached to future Mini-GEMs. It would also be interesting to explore the potential for multiprofessional and interspecialty use of these resources, and how they might integrate with more formal structured training.

Conclusion

The Mini-GEM format provides an effective way of disseminating free, concise, focused, clinical teaching material relating to caring for older patients to a wide audience. The videos were valued by junior doctors due to their accessibility, ease of use on a variety of devices, their perceived credibility and limited duration. Mini-GEMs were viewed in a variety of settings as an adjunct to other learning resources and led to improved confidence in caring for older patients. Further work is needed to explore the optimum duration of the videos to maximize their potential as effective educational resources for a variety of clinical staff that work with older patients.

Acknowledgements

The authors would like to acknowledge the huge efforts and commitment of Kelly Hunt and Peter Brock, who are an integral part of the Association of Elderly Medicine Education. The authors would also like to thank the authors of Mini-GEM content thus far.

References

Barbour, R. S. (2001). Checklists for improving rigour in qualitative research: A case of the tail wagging the dog? British Medical Journal, *322*, 1115–1117. doi:10.1136/bmj.322.7294.1115

Beetham, H., & Sharpe, R. (2007). *Rethinking pedagogy for a digital age: Designing and delivering E-Learning*. London, England: Routledge.

Beyer, A. M. (2011). Improving student presentations: Pecha Kucha and just plain PowerPoint. *Teaching of Psychology*, *38*, 122–126. doi:10.1177/0098628311401588

Bunniss, S., & Kelly, D. R. (2010). Research paradigms in medical education research. *Medical Education*, *44*, 358–366. doi:10.1111/med.2010.44.issue-4

Cook, D. A. (2010). Twelve tips for evaluating educational programs. *Medical Teacher*, *32*, 296–301. doi:10.3109/01421590903480121

Cook, D. A., Bordage, G., & Schmidt, H. G. (2008). Description, justification and clarification: A framework for classifying the purposes of research in medical education. *Medical Education*, *42*(2), 128–133. doi:10.1111/(ISSN)1365-2923

Cook, D. A., Levinson, A. J., Garside, S., Dupras, D. M., Erwin, P. J., & Montori, V. M. (2008). Internet-based learning in the health professions: A meta-analysis. *Journal of the American Medical Association*, *300*(10), 1181–1196. doi:10.1001/jama.300.10.1181

Daunt, L. A., Umeonusulu, P. I., Gladman, J. R. F., Blundell, A. G., Conroy, S. P., & Gordon, A. L. (2013). Undergraduate teaching in geriatric medicine using computer-aided learning improves student performance in examinations. *Age and Ageing*, *43*, 721–724.

Ellaway, R. (2013). Scholarship in an age of big data. *Medical Teacher*, *35*, 613–615. doi:10.3109/0142159X.2013.819685

Ellaway, R. H., Fink, P., Graves, L., & Campbell, A. (2014). Left to their own devices: Medical learners' use of mobile technologies. *Medical Teacher*, *36*, 130–138. doi:10.3109/0142159X.2013.849800

Eraut, M. (2000). Non-formal learning and tacit knowledge in professional work. *British Journal of Educational Psychology*, *70*, 113–136. doi:10.1348/000709900158001

Eskildsen, M. A. (2010). Review of web-based module to train and assess competency in systems-based practice. *Journal of the American Geriatrics Society*, *58*, 2412–2413. doi:10.1111/j.1532-5415.2010.03167.x

Fisher, J. M., Hunt, K., & Garside, M. J. (2014). Geriatrics for juniors: Tomorrow's geriatricians or another lost tribe? *Journal of the Royal College of Physicians of Edinburgh*, *44*, 106–110. doi:10.4997/JRCPE

Forgie, S. E., Duff, J. P., & Ross, S. (2013). Twelve tips for using Twitter as a learning tool in medical education. *Medical Teacher*, *35*, 8–14. doi:10.3109/0142159X.2012.746448

Gordon, A. L., Blundell, A., Dhesi, J. K., Forrester-Paton, C., Forrester-Paton, J., Mitchell, H. K. … Gladman, J. R. F. (2014). UK medical teaching about ageing is improving but there is still work to be done: The second national survey of undergraduate teaching in ageing and geriatric medicine. *Age and Ageing*, *43*, 293–297. doi:10.1093/ageing/aft207

Lau, K. H. V. (2014). Computer-based teaching module design: Principles derived from learning theories. *Medical Education*, *48*, 247–254. doi:10.1111/medu.2014.48.issue-3

Moffett, J. (2015). Twelve tips for "flipping" the classroom. *Medical Teacher, 37,* 331–336. doi:10.3109/0142159X.2014.943710

Nolan, T. (2011). A smarter way to practise. *British Medical Journal, 342,* d1124.

Oakley, R., Pattinson, J., Goldberg, S., Daunt, L., Samra, R., Masud, T. … Gordon, A. L. (2014). Equipping tomorrow's doctors for the patients of today. *Age and Ageing, 43,* 442–447. doi:10.1093/ageing/afu077

Ramaswamy, R., Leipzig, R. M., Howe, C. L., Sauvigne, K., Usiak, C., & Soriano, R. P. (2015). The portal of geriatrics online education: A 21st-century resource for teaching geriatrics. *Journal of the American Geriatrics Society, 63,* 335–340. doi:10.1111/jgs.2015.63.issue-2

Sandars, J., Patel, R. S., Goh, P. S., Kokatailo, P. K., & Lafferty, N. (2015). The importance of educational theories for facilitating learning when using technology in medical education. *Medical Teacher, 37*(11), 1–4. Advance online publication.

Shaw, G. (2013). Breaking news: Don't call it social media: FOAM and the future of medical education. *Emergency Medicine News, 35,* 1–30.

Topps, D., Helmer, J., & Ellaway, R. (2013). YouTube as a platform for publishing clinical skills training videos. *Academic Medicine, 88,* 192–197. doi:10.1097/ACM.0b013e31827c5352

United Nations. Department of Economic and Social Affairs (2015). *World population prospects: The 2012 revision.* Retrieved from http://esa.un.org/wpp/Excel-Data/population.htm

Wallace, S., Clark, M., & White, J. (2012). 'It's on my iPhone': Attitudes to the use of mobile computing devices in medical education, a mixed-methods study. *BMJ Open, 2,* e001099–e001099. doi:10.1136/bmjopen-2012-001099

Yavner, S. D., Pusic, M. V., Kalet, A. L., Song, H. S., Hopkins, M. A., Nick, M. W., & Ellaway, R. H. (2015). Twelve tips for improving the effectiveness of web-based multimedia instruction for clinical learners. *Medical Teacher, 37,* 239–244. doi:10.3109/0142159X.2014.933202

Young, J. Q., Van Merrienboer, J., Durning, S., & Ten Cate, O. (2014). Cognitive Load Theory: Implications for medical education: AMEE Guide No. 86. *Medical Teacher, 36,* 371–384. doi:10.3109/0142159X.2014.889290

Appendix

Discussion guide for focus group

Themes	Example Question
Introduction	Welcome
	Confidentiality/anonymity
	Audio recording
	Explanation of interview structure
	Invite questions
Icebreaker	
Finding the content	How did you hear about the Mini-GEMs?
Accessing the content	Why did you choose to watch a given Mini-GEM?
	What device do you tend to use to watch the Mini-GEMs?
	When do you tend to watch the Mini-GEMs?
	Where do you tend to watch the Mini-GEMs?
Content Style	Do you have any comments about the style or layout of the Mini-GEMs?
	How about the duration of the Mini-GEMs?
After watching	Did you feel the Mini-GEM(s) you watched enabled you to achieve the learning outcomes?
	Have you been able to apply things from the Mini-GEMs to your job?
	Did you access the further reading resources?
Final Questions	What other topics would you like to see covered by future Mini-GEMs?
	Do you have any suggestions for how we might improve the Mini-GEMs?
Close	Any final questions?
	Reiterate re. confidentiality and anonymity
	Thank participants for their time and help with the project

Resident learning across the full range of core competencies through a transitions of care curriculum

Juliessa M. Pavon, Sandro O. Pinheiro, and Gwendolen T. Buhr

ABSTRACT

The authors developed a Transitions of Care (TOC) curriculum to teach and measure learner competence in performing TOC tasks for older adults. Internal medicine interns at an academic residency program received the curriculum, which consisted of experiential learning, self-study, and small group discussion. Interns completed retrospective pre/post surveys rating their confidence in performing five TOC tasks, qualitative open-ended survey questions, and a self-reflection essay. A subset of interns also completed follow-up assessments. For all five TOC tasks, the interns' confidence improved following completion of the TOC curriculum. Self-confidence persisted for up to 3 months later for some but not all tasks. According to the qualitative responses, the TOC curriculum provided interns with learning experiences and skills integral to performing safe care transitions. The TOC curriculum and a mixed-method assessment approach effectively teaches and measures learner competency in TOC across all six Accreditation Council for Graduate Medical Education competency domains.

Introduction

A transition in care is the movement of a patient between health care practitioners and settings. However, the process is complex and occurs most effectively when accompanied by a conscious set of interventions that ensure coordination and continuity of care (Coleman & Boult, 2003). Transitions of care (TOC) interventions are typically applied to older adults most at risk of health complications resulting from poor quality transitions including fragmented care, increased adverse drug events, and increased rehospitalizations and emergency room visits (Coleman & Boult, 2003; Forster, Clark, & Menard et al., 2004; Forster, Murff, Peterson, Ghandi, & Bates, 2003, 2005). A critical component to ensuring successful TOC for vulnerable older adults is quality education for health professionals about care transitions (Aiyer, Kukreja, & Ibrahim-Ali, 2009; Coleman, 2003; Green et al., 2009; Ouchida, LoFaso, Capello, Ramsaroop, & Reid, 2009).

Medical residents, at the front line of care transitions, must be able to perform safe care transitions. The Accreditation Council for Graduate Medical Education (ACGME) supports curriculum development in care transitions for physician trainees (ACGME, 2016; Green et al., 2009). The ACGME's (2016) six core competencies of patient care, medical knowledge, practice-based learning and improvement, interpersonal communication skills, professionalism, and systems-based practice provide a framework for the education and evaluation of trainees. However, few analyses of TOC curricula for medical residents have assessed how effectively these competencies are learned.

As a subsequent step to the development of core competencies, the ACGME created Milestones to evaluate a trainee's progress toward independent practice. To achieve the Milestone on TOC, trainees are expected to show an ability to coordinate care within and across healthcare settings (ACGME, 2015). The ACGME (2014) also created the Clinical Learning Environment Review (CLER) program to evaluate medical resident learning environments and to ensure physician education on patient safety and high-quality care in six focus areas including care transitions. Further, graduating medical students are expected to achieve a minimum level of competence in safe discharge planning, as outlined by the Minimum Geriatrics Competencies for Medical Students (Leipzig et al., 2009). Building on these efforts, the Minimum Geriatrics Competencies for Internal Medicine and Family Medicine Residents were established to further define a minimum but uniform expectation of competency in the geriatrics domain of TOC (Williams et al., 2010). Quality curricula are required to create clinical environments in which medical residents can demonstrate competency in TOC, and these curricula will be highly valuable to programs undergoing ACGME evaluations.

Recognizing this need for quality education on care transitions, we implemented a TOC curriculum to teach internal medicine interns the elements of an evidence-based intervention that has been shown to reduce adverse events during care transitions (Coleman et al., 2004). The goals of this curriculum were (1) greater competence of learners in performing TOC tasks and (2) an increased awareness of the vulnerability of older adults during the TOC process. Results are presented from a mixed-methods evaluation of that curriculum, which uses quantitative and qualitative learner self-assessment and reflection to assess medical intern confidence, attitudes, and knowledge about TOC concepts.

Method

Participants and setting

All internal medicine interns from an academic medical center's Internal Medicine Residency Program were required to complete the TOC curriculum during their geriatric rotation. All medical interns who participated in the residency program's TOC curriculum from 2008 to 2012 completed the learner assessments described below and were eligible for analysis in this study. The geriatrics rotation was a 4-week block rotation that included time at the University Hospital consult service, the comprehensive geriatric assessment clinic, and the Veterans Affair community living center. Additional experiences allowed interns to learn the depth and breadth of geriatric medicine; these included the osteoporosis clinic, the memory disorders clinic, a skilled nursing facility, the primary care clinic in a continuing care retirement community, hospice home visits, and geriatric psychiatry. At each site, the interns interacted with geriatric fellows and faculty as their preceptors. To our knowledge, prior to this curriculum on TOC, there was no existing teaching program.

Curriculum description

The TOC curriculum was based on the Four Pillars of Care Transitions intervention activities (Medication Self-Management, Use of a Dynamic Patient-Centered Record, Primary Care and Specialist Follow-Up, Knowledge of Red Flags) (Coleman et al., 2004), a well-established model that addressed the objectives of our curriculum. Medical interns were assigned to a patient and saw this patient both in the hospital setting (initial encounter) and in the patient's home setting after discharge (follow-up encounter). The selected hospitalized patients were typically from an institution-affiliated Continuing Care Retirement Community. Patients, selected from general medicine or surgical wards, across admission diagnoses and disease severity, were cognitively intact, able to provide a medical history, and expected to stay in the hospital 3 to 5 days. The medical interns (1) coached the patient through a care transition, (2) compiled a medication record collaboratively with the patient by considering the prehospital and posthospital medications, and (3) used a specific tool to identify medication discrepancies [http://caretransi tions.org] (Coleman, n.d.). In addition to the Four Pillars, our TOC curriculum required that the interns evaluate functional status and assess patient equipment or rehabilitation needs.

The instructional strategies used in the TOC curriculum included (1) experiential learning, which involved interns seeing the patient in the hospital and following him/her through a transition, as well as reconciling their medications; (2) self-study of an assigned article (Coleman, Parry, Chalmers, & Min, 2006) that provided a foundation on TOC principles; (3) small-group discussions led by faculty physician educators (with two to four fellow learners) to facilitate debriefing and processing of the experience and to provide an opportunity to address any clinical questions or concerns; and (4) self-reflection through essay writing (Figure 1).

Learner assessment

The learners completing the TOC curriculum were assessed using a mixed-methods approach. Researchers agree that this approach generally yields a more authentic assessment of an educational intervention (Shulman, 1988) and a more holistic, valid picture of the impact of a program compared to either quantitative or qualitative methods alone. In this case, learner assessment consisted of surveys containing quantitative Likert-type scale questions and qualitative open-ended questions, as well as a separate qualitative self-reflection essay. The procedure for this mixed-method assessment strategy is included in Figure 1.

Postcurriculum survey

Immediately after participation in the curriculum, interns anonymously completed a five-item quantitative retrospective pre/post self-efficacy survey rating their confidence in performing TOC tasks before and after completion of the TOC curriculum. These survey items, derived from the objectives of the curriculum, asked learners to self-assess their confidence in ability to (1) identify potential threats to a well-executed transition, (2) anticipate consequences of a poorly executed transition, (3) address changes in functional status, (4) compile pre- and post-hospital medication records, and (5) evaluate medication

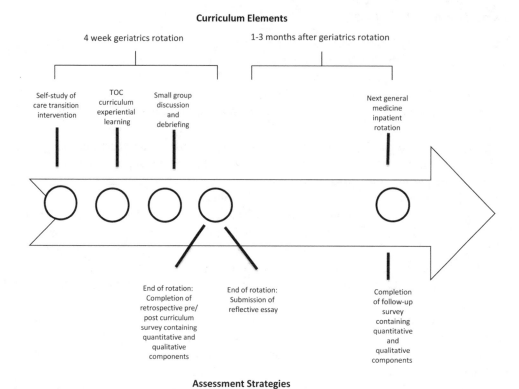

Figure 1. Illustration of the transitions of care curriculum elements and assessment procedure. *Note.* TOC = Transitions of Care.

discrepancies. Confidence in performing each skill was measured using a Likert-type scale ranging from 1 to 5 (1 = *no confidence*, 5 = *completely confident*).

The postcurriculum survey also included two open-ended, short-answer questions: (1) What was the most valuable aspect of this experience for you? and (2) As a result of this activity what will you change about your practice?

Self-reflection essay

Before the end of the geriatrics rotation, learners submitted a self-reflection essay with the only instruction or prompt to write a one-page-or-less reflection on the TOC experience. The purpose of the essay was to evaluate learner attitudes and the influence of the TOC curriculum on clinical practice in a qualitative manner.

Follow-up survey

The follow-up survey was administered as a one-time assessment to provide a report on the success and the sustainable impact of the TOC curriculum on medical intern confidence in performing TOC tasks. Follow-up data, therefore, was collected only on a subset of medical interns participating in the TOC curriculum (intern class 2009–2010) who were selected using convenience sampling. In addition to completing the postcurriculum survey immediately after participation in the TOC curriculum, this sample of interns completed an anonymous follow-up self-efficacy survey following completion of a subsequent general medicine rotation, a point at which the opportunity to apply the learned skills was expected to be highest (range 1–3 months post-TOC curriculum). This follow-up survey assessed confidence in currently performing the five TOC tasks using the same Likert-type scale as in the postcurriculum survey. To evaluate learners' perceived impact of the TOC curriculum on their clinical practice three open-ended questions were included: (1) What aspects of the transition experience were most helpful in informing your practice today? (2) What aspect of the TOC skills have you maintained in your current practice? and (3) As a result of this activity, how has your practice changed?

Quantitative analysis

Means and standard deviations were calculated for each retrospective pre- and postsurvey item to examine the distribution of the data with respect to confidence. The Wilcoxon signed-rank test was used for pairwise comparisons of confidence scores on the pre- and postsurvey items. For a subset of medical interns, comparisons between confidence scores from the postsurvey items on the postcurriculum survey and from the follow-up survey were made at the group level because surveys were anonymous. A paired-sample t test to evaluate the change in the total mean score of confidence ratings between these two groups was performed separately for each task. The data were analyzed using R version 2.15.1 (R Core Team, 2012). This project was approved under exempt status by the institution's Institutional Review Board.

Qualitative analyses

A three-member faculty team composed of two geriatricians and a PhD educator performed qualitative analyses of the (1) postcurriculum open-ended survey questions, (2) reflective essay, and (3) follow-up open-ended survey questions. The aim of these analyses was to determine themes of TOC concepts and skills learned during the rotation. Two authors analyzed postcurriculum open-ended survey questions, and a third author performed verification of coding. Two authors each read 10 reflective essays independently and met to compare and achieve consensus on coding. After consensus was reached, subsequent essays were divided among the three authors for a separate analysis. One author read and analyzed follow-up surveys and the two other authors verified them. Themes from the open-ended survey questions and essays were matched to the ACGME core competencies. Authors also recorded quotations that illustrated the learning themes for the three qualitative assessment strategies.

Results

All internal medicine interns who participated in the residency program's geriatric medicine TOC Experience from 1/2008 to 6/2012 were eligible for this analysis. A total of 111 interns, representing multiple intern classes, were eligible and all completed the postcurriculum self-evaluation survey retrospectively rating their confidence in their ability to complete TOC tasks pre and post completion of the TOC curriculum. Eighty-nine interns completed the reflective essay. Thirty-eight interns from one intern class were selected to complete the long-term follow-up survey during the period from 2/2010 to 11/2010, and 74% ($n = 28$) completed this survey.

For the postcurriculum quantitative survey items, confidence scores between the retrospective pre- and postcurriculum self-ratings increased for all five tasks. On the 5-point rating scale, the average overall precurriculum confidence score was 3.05. The interns were least confident in their abilities to address change in function (2.74) and to identify potential threats to well-executed transitions (2.83). Following completion of the curriculum, interns' confidence in their ability to perform TOC tasks improved an average of 1.20 points on a 5-point scale. The greatest improvement (+1.40) was seen in ability to evaluate medication discrepancies, followed by ability to identify potential threats to a well-executed care transition (+1.34). At 1 to 3 months following completion of the TOC curriculum, there was no significant change in mean scores regarding confidence in ability to anticipate consequences, compile medications, or evaluate medication discrepancies; however, there was a decrease in scores for confidence in ability to identify threats to well-executed care transitions (post 4.24/follow-up 4.00; $p = .043$) and address changes in functional status (post 3.97/follow-up 3.63; $p = .049$) (Table 1). Nevertheless, all follow-up confidence ratings were higher than the retrospective pre-curriculum confidence ratings on each TOC task.

Qualitative methods were used to assess knowledge, attitudes, and self-reported behaviors about TOC. The postcurriculum short-answer results are summarized in Table 2. Not surprisingly, the interns commented on the value of the practical experience of seeing the patient's home living environment, appreciating the patient perspective, and empowering the patient and caregivers. The interns also mentioned the importance of medication reconciliation, communication with the patient and primary care physician (PCP), and the patient's functional status and equipment needs. In addition, the interns discussed the knowledge they gained about long-term care settings, patient functional status, and the

Table 1. Confidence in ability to accomplish transitions of care tasks[a].

Question: How confident are you in your ability to:	Pre/post curriculum surveys (2008–2012)			Post-curriculum/follow-up surveys (2010)		
	Pretest mean (SD) N = 111	Posttest mean (SD) N = 111	p value	Postcurriculum survey, posttest mean (SD) N = 38	Follow-up mean (SD) N = 28	p value[b]
Identify potential threats to a well-executed transition between sites of care	2.83 (0.58)	4.17 (0.39)	< 0.001	4.24 (0.49)	4.00 (0.38)	0.043
Anticipate the consequences of poorly executed care transitions	3.17 (0.89)	4.26 (0.54)	< 0.001	4.29 (0.61)	4.07 (0.54)	0.424
Address changes in physical function and new equipment needs	2.74 (0.81)	3.91 (0.51)	< 0.001	3.97 (0.68)	3.63 (0.74)[c]	0.049
Compile a medication record collaboratively with a patient or caregiver considering the pre-hospital and post-hospital medications	3.61 (0.94)	4.65 (0.49)	< 0.001	4.49 (0.69)[d]	4.68 (0.48)	0.264
Evaluate for medication discrepancies using specific tools (e.g. Medication Discrepancy Tool)	2.95 (1.09)	4.35 (0.58)	< 0.001	4.29 (0.77)	4.54 (0.58)	0.326

[a] Five-point scale where 1 = no confidence at all and 5 = completely confident.
[b] p Value reflects difference in means only between post- and follow-up self-confidence ratings.
[c] Missing = 1 response.
[d] Missing = 1 response.

Table 2. Postcurriculum survey short-answer qualitative findings mapped to Accreditation Council for Graduate Medical Education (ACGME) core competencies.[a]

Themes	Sample supporting quotes	ACGME core competencies
The patient's perspective and home living environment	"You can learn so much more about how a patient is doing by seeing them at home." "It is helpful to see firsthand how difficult transitions can be for patients and families."	Patient Care Systems-based Practice
Gaining knowledge about LTC	"The patient's biggest concern about the transition may not be the physician's." "Seeing a nursing home; understanding what they do and don't do there." "Seeing a nursing home and being aware of who is receiving the patient after discharge; i.e. there isn't a physician waiting to receive the patient."	Medical Knowledge Systems-based Practice
Communication with patients and caregivers	"More focus placed on patient education and accurate discharge instructions, and anticipating needs of patient and family." "Meeting the patient and her family. I found it really helpful and invigorating to see how a little time spent on their issues could relieve a tremendous amount of fear, anxiety, and pain." "It is really eye-opening how poorly we communicate our reasons for doing certain treatments, why we start certain drugs."	Interpersonal and Communication Skills Professionalism Practice-based Learning and Improvement
Functional status and equipment needs	"It is important to understand their prior level of functioning and if their new needs are appropriate for their prior level of care." "Make deeper evaluation of patient functional needs."	Medical Knowledge Patient Care
Learning about transitions of care	"Realizing this is a real problem." "Being made aware of issues that occur during transitions. I had never really thought much about it." "Learning aspects of transitions of care to aid in my understanding of discharge planning."	Medical Knowledge Systems-based Practice
Empowerment of patients and caregivers	"Will definitely encourage patients to be more active in their own care, especially during transitions." "Learn to empower the patient to know meds and ask questions post discharge regarding reaching goals and returning to baseline."	Patient Care Professionalism Practice-based Learning and Improvement

Notes. LTC = long-term care; PCP = primary care physician.

[a] Quotes are in response to the questions: "What was the most valuable aspect of this experience for you?" and "As a result of this activity what will you change about your practice?" mapped to ACGME core competencies.

TOC process. These learner responses mapped to the ACGME core competencies of patient care, interpersonal and communication skills, professionalism, medical knowledge, and systems-based practice (Table 2).

Table 3 is a summary of the reflection essay themes. The interns wrote about the factors supporting successful TOC, which separated into five categories: (1) communication with and education of patients and caregivers, (2) communication with PCP and other providers, (3) patient empowerment, (4) support from caregivers, and (5) other resources. Interns also commented on barriers to successful transitions, which also divided into five categories: (1) break-down in communication between settings, (2) break-down in communication among the medical team and the patient, (3) patient lack of involvement with and knowledge of his or her health conditions or medications, (4) lack of resources, and (5) system complexity. These themes matched to competencies in patient care, interpersonal and communication skills, professionalism, practice-based learning and improvement, and systems-based practice (Table 3).

The interns also gained appreciation for aspects of geriatrics care such as elders' vulnerability during transitions. One intern wrote:

> Change is difficult. Multiple changes are even worse. And multiple changes without understanding simply invite disaster. Yet, with full knowledge of these challenges, we physicians discharge patients every day from the hospital and from clinic with new diagnoses, new disabilities, multiple medication changes, unknown obstacles at home, and minimal information to prepare them for such transitions. The risk for substantial patient morbidity and mortality is high.

Finally, there were essays that clearly reflected value and attitude changes in the intern, a new appreciation of the patient perspective, and commitments to change his or her practice going forward. One intern wrote about the patient's perspective:

> I had never really considered the confusion or difficulty that could arise from a hospital stay or from a move to a skilled nursing facility or returning home.... It was the first time I had asked a patient about how they felt about leaving the hospital and if they had concerns. I wasn't anticipating the response. I thought she would be happy to be going home, not apprehensive of what lay ahead for her.

Other interns reflected on the importance of focusing on the transition. One wrote:

> I believe it is a common sentiment by many physicians that "as soon as the patient leaves my care or my sight, it is no longer my problem." This experience has taught me that what goes on after hospitalization is more important than what transpired during hospitalization.

The short-answer results in the follow-up survey reflected similar themes as the short-answer and reflection essays that were completed immediately following the curriculum activity (the appendix). In response to the question "What aspects of the transitions experience (curriculum) were most helpful in informing your practice today?", the interns highlighted the value of the experiential learning nature of the activity and through this were able to learn about the importance of medication education and reconciliation, communication with patients and caregivers, support from caregivers, appreciation of the patient's perspective, and evaluation of functional status and equipment needs. When asked how an understanding of the TOC curriculum changed their practice, many interns commented that they became more aware of medication changes and were better at

Table 3. Reflection essay qualitative findings related to transitions of care mapped to Accreditation Council for Graduate Medical Education (ACGME) core competencies.

Theme	Categories	Sample supporting quotes	ACGME core competencies
Factors supporting successful transitions	Communication with and education of patients and caregivers	"It became clear from this that simply asking patients if they understood their instructions or had any questions was not sufficient. …Rather, I now realize that I need to have patients explain back to me why they are taking what they are taking and any important instructions. I need to give them more opportunity to ask questions, and even tell them that I expect some questions, and give them a day or two to think about what they would like to ask. Further, for patients with complicated instructions or significant changes during their hospital stay, a simple phone call within several days of discharge to follow-up with the patient and answer any questions that may have arisen after leaving the hospital may help prevent medication confusion and error and prevent unnecessary re-hospitalizations."	Interpersonal and Communication Skills Practice-based Learning and Improvement
	Communication with PCP and other providers	"The way that this experience will change my practice is to communicate with other providers on admission and discharge, particularly for patients where significant changes were made or had a complicated hospital course."	Interpersonal and Communication Skills Practice-based learning and Improvement
	Patient empowerment	"The empowering of patients is critical as we cannot control the commitment of all providers to make these transitions as smooth as possible." "Despite best efforts, mistakes are made, and empowering patients to take ownership of their medication list and to ask questions about any discrepancies or confusing instructions provides an important system of additional checks to ensure that transitions occur as smoothly as possible."	Interpersonal and Communication Skills Practice-based Learning and Improvement
	Support from caregivers	"One point of emphasis should also go towards getting family members, caretakers, or friends more involved in the discharge planning as they can, in essence, serve as a patient's coach by fulfilling the role of assisting with medications and follow-up appointments."	Systems-based practice Interpersonal and Communication Skills
	Other resources	"And while I left this patient reassured that he would handle his medical transition gracefully, I also left with increased concern about other patients headed home without his resources." "A common electronic medical record system would benefit both patient and provider."	Systems-based practice Professionalism

Barriers to Successful Transitions		
Break-down in communication between settings	"It became obvious that the transfer of records from the nursing home to the … emergency room and then to the primary team was a process with significant fallibility.… Frequently records handled in the emergency room are not communicated to the inpatient team or the inpatient team does not pursue these records."	Interpersonal and Communication Skills Systems-based practice
Break-down in communication among the medical team and the patient	"Ever since she had come to the hospital she felt that she had lost that independence. She was unsure of not only the changes that had been made to her medication regimen but also about the care she was receiving. She was upset that the steps of her care were not being explained to her. As she stated: 'It's as if the team is talking over me, not to me.'"	Interpersonal and Communication Skills
Patient lack of involvement with and knowledge of his/her health condition or medications	"My patient in this experience had a paternalistic view of medicine. He often stated that 'I will do whatever you guys tell me, you are the Doctors'. There was no motivation on his part to get involved and ask questions about his care and why he is receiving certain medications." "Coaching her through the transition from hospital to SNF highlighted the difficulties that elderly patients face in taking an active role in their healthcare amidst changing functional status, changes in medications, and the stress associated with changing environments."	Practice-based Learning and Improvement Patient Care
Lack of resources	"In particular, patients without supportive family, without healthcare literacy, patients with dementia, and patients transitioning to home with minimal supportive care, are all at risk for complications with transitions of care."	Systems-based practice
System complexity	"The medical student or intern may complete the discharge instruction (which the nurse, typically, reads and submits to the patient), but the upper-level resident dictates the STAT discharge summary, which **should** list the same medications as the discharge instructions. At the nursing facility, a nurse often copies by hand the medications listed in the [discharge] summary to the patient's/resident's chart—a process that can introduce another level of potential error."	Systems-based practice

SNF = skilled nursing facility.

communicating these changes to patients at the time of discharge. When asked which TOC skills were maintained in their practice, most interns divulged that they were now more consistent in providing medication education and reconciliation, whereas others wrote about continuing to focus on communication with PCPs. These themes mapped across all six core competencies and most commonly to the domains of patient care, interpersonal and communication skills, and practice-based learning and improvement (the appendix).

Discussion

The number of TOC curricula targeting physician trainees has grown in recent years in direct response to calls from national organizations to improve transitional care education (Buchanan & Besdine, 2011; Coleman & Boult, 2003; Green et al., 2009; Society of Hospital Medicine, 2006). Lacking from the literature are studies that report how well the ACGME (2016) core competencies were learned from existing TOC curricula. In addition, most of the published curricula are brief interventions, utilizing classroom-based strategies, and are designed for large groups (Buchanan & Besdine, 2011). Here we report a TOC curriculum that utilized experiential methods to improve medical intern confidence, knowledge, attitudes, and practice behaviors about TOC; learning was consistent across all six ACGME competencies.

Results suggest that following completion of the TOC curriculum, medical interns were more confident in their ability to identify the strengths and limitations of a successful care transition and also to collect and organize critical information about patient medications and function. These results are consistent with other study findings that suggest that TOC curricula are effective in increasing learner confidence (Bray-Hall, Schmidt, & Aagaard, 2010; Lai, Nye, Bookwalter, Kwan, & Hauer, 2008; Ouchida et al., 2009). However, our learning evaluation strategy differs greatly from prior studies. Retrospective pre/post testing has been shown to provide more accurate and reliable data regarding learners' perceptions when compared to original pretesting; in the former learners are more knowledgeable about the concepts learned and can realistically attribute perceived improvements to the intervention completed (Skeff, Stratos, & Bergen, 1992). A possible limitation though of retrospective pre/post testing is that learners' responses may reflect desired instead of actual improvements. However, a main advantage of retrospective pre/post testing, and the reason we chose it for our design, is that it is a one-time administered test, which saves time for curriculum learners and faculty. This self-assessment approach may be a valuable option for diversifying learner assessment strategies in TOC education interventions (Buchanan & Besdine, 2011).

We also used qualitative assessment strategies to measure learner competency in performing TOC by providing short-answer questions on the postcurriculum survey as well as a self-reflection essay. The advantage of qualitative learner assessment through short-answer questions is that it documents how and why the TOC curriculum works to achieve competency and knowledge in care transitions. A review of self-reflection comments by interns on topics such as communication, patient and caregiver involvement in transitions, and system complexities, revealed learning occurred across all six ACGME core competencies. Additionally, even though other formal geriatrics competencies in TOC (e.g., Minimum Competencies for IM-FM residents) (Williams et al., 2010) were published after this TOC curriculum was developed, learning from our curriculum also map to the Minimum Competencies of (1) recognizing system complexities and (2) communicating key components of a safe discharge including medications, functional status, and follow-up coordination with primary care providers. Although this study did not utilize direct observation of medical residents performing TOC tasks, the results suggest that self-reflection can indirectly capture self-reported behaviors that effectively assess medical resident knowledge as well as ability to perform TOC skills. Self-reflection can be a useful assessment method for other curriculum designs in which direct observation is not feasible.

Through self-reflective written essay, we gained insight into how the medical interns processed the TOC curriculum and why and how they planned to integrate the information learned from the experience. Brief reflective writing exercises have been proposed as a technique to foster self-directed learning skills, encourage humanism, and personalize learning for students (Branch et al., 2001; Stern & Papadakis, 2006). These skills were evident in interns' recounts of enhanced communication and patient involvement, which mapped to core competencies in patient care and practice-based learning and improvement.

There is limited knowledge about the sustainable impact of TOC curricula. Administrators of TOC curricula routinely cite the inability to measure sustainability as a limitation. This study is one of the few studies that examines the influence of a TOC curriculum on follow-up rotations and describes a learner assessment strategy used to capture this information. Results from our follow-up quantitative learner assessments support the sustained impact of the TOC curriculum on provider practice. Responses to short-answer survey questions also qualitatively supported the continued impact of the TOC curriculum on provider practice. Specifically, many learners were transferring new knowledge about medication reconciliation into other clinical practice rotations. However, the failure to retain self-confidence with regard to the identification of threats to a well-executed transition and addressing changes in functional status suggests that additional training in these two areas should be included in future TOC curricula.

The most significant limitation of this study is that we did not directly observe residents performing care transitions. Future curricula should incorporate elements to align with the ACGME CLER program goals of promoting direct learner observation. Other possible methodological limitations include the use of a nonvalidated confidence scale and open-ended questions. One limitation of the follow-up assessment strategy we employed is that within person variation between postcurriculum surveys and follow-up surveys are not evaluable. In addition, concrete conclusions are difficult to reach due to the convenience sampling used. However, despite a short interval between completing the TOC curriculum and completing the follow-up survey, as well as a moderate response rate for follow-up surveys, we achieved theme saturation. Improved self-efficacy strongly predicts academic performance, further supporting this follow-up assessment strategy to demonstrate sustained learning and intention to practice (Pajares, 2002). The evidence of this finding needs to be supported with future larger and random samples of interns. Another possible limitation is generalizability, as the study was conducted at a single medical residency program. We tried to mitigate this by involving all medical interns who completed the geriatrics rotation over multiple academic years.

To better evaluate medical resident training in safe and high-quality TOC, curricula that can map learning to core competencies are needed. Our TOC curriculum content effectively taught interns how to perform safe care transitions, and its robust, mixed-methods learner assessment strategy illustrates the diversity of the learning experience across all six ACGME core competency domains. Curriculum developers can replicate our curriculum and assessment approach in other clinical settings to effectively teach and measure learning across the full range of ACGME core clinical competencies.

Acknowledgments

Authors Sandro O. Pinheiro and Gwendolen T. Buhr contributed equally to this work. The authors would like to thank Mitchell T. Heflin, MD, MHS from Duke University, Division of Geriatrics, for his interpretation of the results and critical review of the manuscript, and Caroline Connor, PhD for her critical review and editing of the manuscript.

Conflicts of interest disclosures

The authors have no conflicts of interests to disclose.

Funding

Funding support came from the Geriatric Academic Career Award 1K01 HP00111 (Buhr) and the Duke Greenfield Chiefs Research Award (Pavon). The funders had no role in the design and conduct of the study; collection, management, analysis, and interpretation of the data; preparation, review, or approval of the manuscript; or decision to submit the manuscript for publication. Portions of this work were conducted while Dr. Pavon was supported by funding from the T. Franklin Williams Scholars Program.

References

Accreditation Council for Graduate Medical Education. (2014). *Clinical learning environment review pathways to excellence*. Retrieved from https://www.acgme.org/acgmeweb/Portals/0/PDFs/CLER/CLER_Brochure.pdf

Accreditation Council for Graduate Medical Education. (2015). The Internal Medicine Milestone Project. Retrieved from http://www.acgme.org/acgmeweb/Portals/0/PDFs/Milestones/InternalMedicineMilestones.pdf

Accreditation Council for Graduate Medical Education. (2016). Common Program Requirements. Retrieved from http://www.acgme.org/acgmeweb/Portals/0/PFAssets/ProgramRequirements/CPRs2013.pdf

Aiyer, M., Kukreja, S., & Ibrahim-Ali, W. (2009). Discharge planning curricula in internal medicine residency programs: A national survey. *Southern Medical Journal, 102,* 795–799.

Branch, W. T., Kern, D., Haidet, P., Weissmann, P., Gracey, C. F., Mitchell, G., & Inui, T. (2001). Teaching the human dimensions of care in clinical settings. *Journal of the American Medical Association, 286,* 1067–1074. doi:10.1001/jama.286.9.1067

Bray-Hall, S., Schmidt, K., & Aagaard, E. (2010). Toward safe hospital discharge: A transitions in care curriculum for medical students. *Journal of General Internal Medicine, 25*(8), 878–881. doi:10.1007/s11606-010-1364-3

Buchanan, I. M., & Besdine, R. W. (2011). A systematic review of curricular interventions teaching transitional care to physicians-in-training and physicians. *Academic Medicine, 86,* 628–639. doi:10.1097/ACM.0b013e318212e36c

Coleman, E. A. (2003). Falling through the cracks: Challenges and opportunities for improving transitional care for persons with continuous complex care needs. *Journal of the American Geriatrics Society, 51,* 549–555. doi:10.1046/j.1532-5415.2003.51185.x

Coleman, E. A. (n.d.). Medication discrepancy tool. Retrieved from http://caretransitions.org/wp-content/uploads/2015/08/MDT.pdf

Coleman, E. A., & Boult, C. (2003). Improving the quality of transitional care for persons with complex care needs. *Journal of the American Geriatrics Society, 51,* 556–557. doi:10.1046/j.1532-5415.2003.51186.x

Coleman, E. A., Parry, C., Chalmers, S., & Min, S. J. (2006). The care transitions intervention: Results of a randomized controlled trial. *Archives of Internal Medicine, 166,* 1822–1828. doi:10.1001/archinte.166.17.1822

Coleman, E. A., Smith, J. D., Frank, J. C., Min, S. J., Parry, C., & Kramer, A. M. (2004). Preparing patients and caregivers to participate in care delivered across settings: The Care Transitions Intervention. *Journal of the American Geriatrics Society, 52,* 1817–1825. doi:10.1111/jgs.2004.52.issue-11

Forster, A. J., Clark, H. D., Menard, A., Dupuis, N., Chernish, R., Chandok, N., Khan, A., van Walraven, C. (2004). Adverse events among medical patients after discharge from hospital. *CMAJ: Canadian Medical Association Journal = Journal De L'association Medicale Canadienne, 170,* 345–349.

Forster, A. J., Murff, H. J., Peterson, J. F., Ghandi, T. K., & Bates, D. W. (2003). The incidence and severity of adverse events affecting patients after discharge from the hospital. *Annals of Internal Medicine, 138,* 161–167. doi:10.7326/0003-4819-138-3-200302040-00007

Forster, A. J., Murff, H. J., Peterson, J. F., Ghandi, T. K., & Bates, D. W. (2005). Adverse drug events occurring following hospital discharge. *Journal of General Internal Medicine, 20,* 317–323. doi:10.1111/j.1525-1497.2005.30390.x

Green, M. L., Aagaard, E. M., Caverzagie, K. J., Chick, D. A., Holmboe, E., Kane, G. ... Iobst, W. (2009). Charting the road to competence: Developmental milestones for internal medicine residency training. *Journal of Graduate Medical Education, 1,* 5–20. doi:10.4300/01.01.0003

Lai, C. J., Nye, H. E., Bookwalter, T., Kwan, A., & Hauer, K. E. (2008). Postdischarge follow-up visits for medical and pharmacy students on an inpatient medicine clerkship. *Journal of Hospital Medicine: an Official Publication of the Society of Hospital Medicine, 3,* 20–27. doi:10.1002/(ISSN)1553-5606

Leipzig, R. M., Granville, L., Simpson, D., Brownell Anderson, M., Sauvigne, K., & Soriano, R. P. (2009). Keeping granny safe on July 1: A consensus on minimum geriatrics competencies for graduating medical students. *Academic Medicine, 84,* 604–610. doi:10.1097/ACM.0b013e31819fab70

Ouchida, K., LoFaso, V. M., Capello, C. F., Ramsaroop, S., & Reid, M. C. (2009). Fast forward rounds: An effective method for teaching medical students to transition patients safely across care settings. *Journal of the American Geriatrics Society, 57,* 910–917. doi:10.1111/jgs.2009.57.issue-5

Pajares, F. (2002). *Self-efficacy beliefs in academic contexts: An outline.* Retrieved from http://www.uky.edu/~eushe2/Pajares/efftalk.html

R Core Team. (2012). *R: A language and environment for statistical computing.* Vienna, Austria: R Foundation for Statistical Computing. ISBN 3-900051-07-0. Retrieved from http://www.R-project.org/

Shulman, L. S. (1988). A union of insufficiencies: Strategies for teacher assessment in a period of educational reform. *Educational Leadership, 46,* 36–41.

Skeff, K. M., Stratos, G. A., & Bergen, M. R. (1992). Evaluation of a medical faculty development program: A comparison of traditional pre/post and retrospective pre/post self-assessment ratings. *Evaluation & the Health Professions, 15,* 350–366. doi:10.1177/016327879201500307

Society of Hospital Medicine. (2006). The core competencies in hospital medicine: A framework for curriculum development by the Society of Hospital Medicine. *Journal of Hospital Medicine: an Official Publication of the Society of Hospital Medicine, 1*(Suppl 1), 2–95.

Stern, D. T., & Papadakis, M. (2006). The developing physician—Becoming a professional. *New England Journal of Medicine, 355,* 1794–1799. doi:10.1056/NEJMra054783

Williams, B. C., Warshaw, G., Fabiny, A. R., Lundebjerg, N., Medina-Walpole, A., Sauvigne, K. ... Leipzig, R. M. (2010). Medicine in the 21st century: Recommended essential geriatrics competencies for internal medicine and family medicine residents. *Journal of Graduate Medical Education, 2,* 373–383. doi:10.4300/JGME-D-10-00065.1

Appendix

Follow-up survey short-answer qualitative findings mapped to Accreditation Council for Graduate Medical Education (ACGME) Core Competencies

Themes	Quotes	ACGME core competencies
Question 1: What aspects of the transitions experience (curriculum) were most helpful in informing your practice today?		
Experiential learning	"Practical experience addressing the issues with transitions of care." "Having the opportunity to think about patients through their transition was useful… this isn't something we usually have the chance to do."	Practice-based Learning and Improvement
Medication education and reconciliation	"Evaluating for potential hazards (i.e. medication issues) patients face when transitioning from the hospital to another facility or home." "Showing how much time can sometimes be required to reconcile medications, i.e. when patients are elderly and on multiple meds and memory problems…"	Patient Care Medical Knowledge
Communication with patients, caregivers, and PCPs	"I believe it makes my discharge instructions much more explicit when I am sending persons home from the hospital."	Interpersonal and Communication Skills Practice-based Learning and Improvement
Support from caregivers and other resources	"Understanding the patient's concerns about leaving the hospital and going wherever they may be going, and identifying social support mechanisms."	Patient Care Interpersonal and Communication Skills
The patient's perspective and home living environment	"This exercise was most helpful from an enlightening stand point. It was interesting and beneficial to view the transition from hospital to home/other from a different perspective which has allowed me to pay more attention to details that I otherwise would overlook." "Meeting the patient in both the inpatient as well as their home environment."	Patient Care Practice-based Learning and Improvement
Functional status and equipment needs	"Looking at changes in physical function and the need for home adjustments/equipment. Geriatric population is different than the normal adult population, more specific things that need to be addressed like fall risk, home safety, ADLs."	Patient Care Medical Knowledge
Question 2: As a result of this activity how has your practice changed?		
Medication education and reconciliation	"I am more cognizant of the potential detrimental effects to the patient from not properly reconciling medications or explaining medication changes upon discharge." "I am more conscious of medication changes and patient education for medication changes at time of discharge."	Patient Care Interpersonal and Communication Skills Practice-based Learning and Improvement

(Continued)

(Continued).

Themes	Quotes	ACGME core competencies
Support from caregivers and other resources	"I now ask more questions about my patients living situation and support systems, especially for those with chronic/advanced disease."	Patient Care Interpersonal and Communication Skills
Question 3: What aspects of the TOC skills have you maintained in your practice?		
Medication education and reconciliation	"Vigilance about medication reconciliation as I have seen errors carried over when info is taken from the chart and not verified with the patient." "I have made consistent efforts to write out medicine regimens and go over with my patient's their meds rather than only letting the nurse read my sheet."	Patient Care Interpersonal and Communication Skills Practice-based Learning and Improvement Systems-based Practice
Communication with patients, caregivers, and PCPs	"I try to do very careful med reconciliation and outline any changes, deletions, or additions to the patient and family, including rationale. Obviously, I sometimes do better at this than others, but I am more mindful of it." "Focusing more on contacting primary physicians with paperwork."	Patient Care Interpersonal and Communication Skills Professionalism Systems-based Practice

Note. PCP = primary care physician; ADL = activities of daily living.

Development and preliminary evaluation of the resident coordinated-transitional care (RC-TraC) program: A sustainable option for transitional care education

Elizabeth Chapman, Alexis Eastman, Andrea Gilmore-Bykovskyi, Bennett Vogelman, and Amy Jo Kind

ABSTRACT

Older adults often face poor outcomes when transitioning from hospital to home. Although physicians play a key role in overseeing transitions, there is a lack of practice-based educational programs that prepare resident physicians to manage care transitions of older adults. An educational intervention to provide residents with real-life transitional care practice was therefore developed—Resident-coordinated Transitional Care (RC-TraC). RC-TraC adapted the evidence-based Coordinated-Transitional Care (C-TraC) nurse role for residents, providing opportunities to follow patients during the peri-hospital period without additional costs to the residency program. Between July 2010 and June 2013, 31 internal medicine residents participated in RC-TraC, caring for 721 patients. RC-TraC has been a sustainable, low-cost, practice-based education experience that is recognized as transitional care education by residents and continues in operation to this day. RC-TraC is a promising option for geriatric-based transitional care education of resident physicians and could also be adapted for nonphysician learners.

Introduction

Older adults are at risk for a range of negative outcomes after hospital discharge, including medication discrepancies (Coleman, Smith, Raha, & Min, 2005), lack of appropriate follow-up (Coleman, 2003), unnecessary emergency room visits, and rehospitalization (Coleman & Berenson, 2004). Health care systems are often ill equipped to handle the complex needs of older adults with multiple chronic conditions as they leave the hospital (Hirschman, Shaid, McCauley, Pauly, & Naylor, 2015). With higher rates of multimorbidity (Gerteis et al., 2014) and of complicating problems like frailty and cognitive impairment, geriatric patients are particularly vulnerable to the health care system gaps that lead to complicated transitions (Hirschman et al., 2015).

Although physicians play a key role in hospital discharge processes, formal instruction during residency training on providing care to elderly patients as they leave the hospital is limited. The

Accreditation Council for Graduate Medical Education (ACGME, 2015; Riebschleger & Philibert, 2011 requires residency programs to provide transitional care instructionand, and models for such education have proliferated recently (Buchanan & Besdine, 2011). Specific educational standards are vague, however, and most existing programs rely on lecture-based tools (Buchanan & Besdine, 2011). Data suggest that this prevailing structure—didactics without skill practice opportunities—does not effectively change physician behaviors (Forsetlund et al., 2009). Further, though more transitional care education models have emerged in the literature, little data exist regarding feasibility or sustainability.

To address these gaps, a geriatric-based transitional care educational program for internal medicine residents called RC-TraC (Resident-coordinated Transitional Care) was developed from an existing rotation previously lacking a transitional care curriculum. A successful nurse-led transitional care program called Coordinated Transitional Care (C-TraC) served as the model for RC-TraC (Kind et al., 2012). In previous testing, C-TraC decreased 30-day rehospitalizations by one third and estimated costs by more than $1,200 per patient (Kind, 2012). C-TraC itself has been sustainable, continues in operation to this day, and has disseminated to multiple other sites. Keeping RC-TraC cost neutral for the residency program was also critical to ensure that it, like C-TraC, was sustainable and feasible. The following details the adaptation of the clinical C-TraC program to create a transitional care educational experience for residents.

Method

Setting and participants

This midwestern academic internal medicine residency program includes rotations in three hospital settings, including an 87-bed tertiary care Veterans Affairs (VA) hospital. The residency program comprises 87 trainees, of whom 31 have VA-based primary care clinics. The remaining 56 trainees see patients in university-affiliated clinics. Only residents with VA primary care clinics participate in the RC-TraC rotation, rotating once during intern year and at least once thereafter. The VA hospital sees approximately 4,400 admissions annually, drawing patients across three states. C-TraC-eligible veterans have an average age of 75 years and are medically complex (Kind, 2012).

RC-TraC program description

RC-TraC evolved from C-TraC, a protocolized, nurse-led geriatric-based transitional care program employing inpatient team integration, in-hospital visits with patients/families, and intensive phone-based contacts with transitioning patients/families in the posthospital period. C-TraC utilizes basic tenets of transitional care in its protocols, including patient and caregiver empowerment, medication reconciliation, development of individualized, patient-specific "red flags," coordination of follow-up, and provision of direct contacts for postdischarge concerns (Coleman & Chalmers, 2006)

RC-TraC launched on July 1, 2010, growing from an existing 4-week "urgent care" rotation where residents saw patients with pressing medical issues in a clinic (Figure 1). To incorporate transitional care education, a team of educators, residents, and transitional care experts

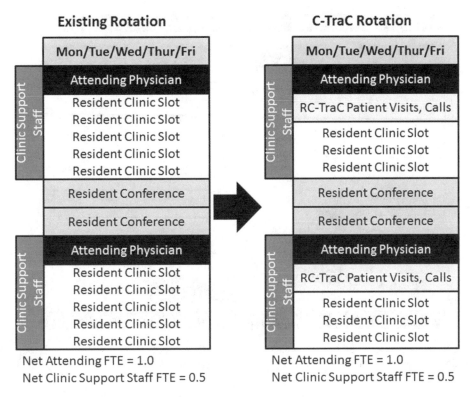

Figure 1. Incorporation of resident-coordinated transitional care (RC-TraC) into existing clinic rotation structures.

adapted C-TraC protocols (Kind, 2012) via an iterative process so resident physicians could assume the role of C-TraC nurses.

RC-TraC follows protocols (Figure 2) nearly identical to C-TraC (Kind, 2012). Residents meet eligible hospitalized patients in person before discharge and begin the process of patient education and empowerment. They elicit concerns, provide a list of individualized "red flags" that should prompt medical attention, write down a direct telephone number the patient can use to ask questions or share concerns, and verify if the patient can attend follow-up appointments. If issues arise, residents serve as liaisons to the inpatient team, seeking solutions before discharge. Additionally, the resident verifies the patient's contact information and schedules a time to contact the patient by telephone within 72 hours after discharge. The encounter is documented in the electronic medical record using the C-TraC program template notes.

Thereafter, residents and patients communicate via telephone until program completion. During the contacts, residents utilize a protocolized, scripted question list and document in C-TraC note templates. The first posthospital contact includes a detailed, patient-led medication reconciliation, review of "red flags," and inquiry about other concerns. Residents also ensure the patient can attend follow-up appointments. Subsequent calls follow standard C-TraC protocols, with regular review of "red flags." Staff physicians who oversaw residents in the former clinic rotation now act as attendings for RC-TraC, guiding development of discharge plans for RC-TraC patients, and assisting in triage of concerns noted during

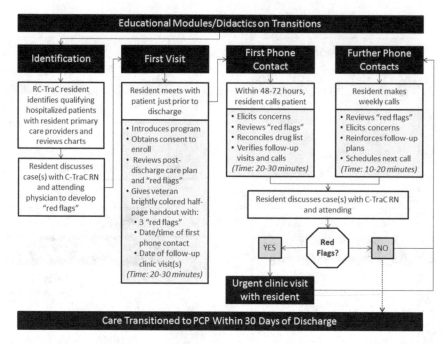

Figure 2. Resident-coordinated transitional care (RC-TraC) protocol. FTE = C-TraC = Coordinated-Transitional Care; RN = registered nurse; PCP = primary care physician.

contacts. When patients reach 30 days postdischarge, see their primary care providers, or mutually agree no additional follow-up is necessary, they discharge from RC-TraC.

In addition to providing direct transitional care for patients, residents participate in didactic sessions on transitional care, system considerations, and health policy during the rotation through online learning modules, assigned reading, and narrated presentations (see the appendix).

Measures/analysis

RC-TraC residents maintain a clinical spreadsheet tracking enrollment volumes. The number of participating residents for July 2010 through June 2013 was also calculated. Additionally, a 24-item survey of residents conducted during May and June 2013 included one question addressing recognition of transitional care education. The question asked, "Have you had formal training during residency regarding transitions of care? (Yes/No)." Because only residents with VA primary care clinics rotate in RC-TraC, residents with university-based clinics served as a convenient comparison group. Item frequencies for the ordinal survey question from RC-TraC participants and nonparticipants were compared, with the difference assessed using a chi-square test. p Values were two-sided. Statistical analysis was performed using Stata 12 software (StataCorp., College Station, TX). The university hospital's Institutional Review Board and the VA Research and Development Committee deemed this project "not research" and did not require participant informed consent.

Results

Adaptation of C-TraC to accommodate resident learners

Adapting the clinical RN role in C-TraC to one appropriate for resident education required key alterations to account for differences in training background, practice scope, and supervision requirements (Table 1). Unlike physician education, nursing training often emphasizes patient education and creation of patient-specific care plans. Formal discharge processes rely heavily on nursing for discharge education, and telephone triage is a well-established nursing role. Residents are only peripherally involved in education of patients at discharge and rarely have front-line contact over the telephone with recently discharged patients.

As a result, resident physicians required coaching from experienced transitional care nurses from C-TraC and attending physicians. For each patient, residents independently developed a list of "red flag" symptoms and received input from a C-TraC RN and attending physician with specific focus on the use of patient-friendly terminology and prioritization of symptoms most likely to suggest clinical deterioration. These transition coaches also helped triage patients' concerns, schedule clinic visits, and facilitate hand-offs to incoming residents at the end of the 4-week rotation. The coaching role ensured patients' specific risks for readmission were addressed and improved care continuity while providing the supervision for residents expected in training programs.

Differences in practice scope between physicians and nurses provided new opportunities for in-person contact with patients after discharge in RC-TraC. C-TraC registered nurses (RNs) have extensive telephone contact with patients, but resident physicians can also see patients in follow-up clinic visits, connecting discharge plans of care, with outpatient management. RC-TraC residents thus provide additional in-person outpatient care to their colleague's patients rather than just alerting colleagues to problems. With these changes, RC-TraC still maintained a high degree of fidelity to the original C-TraC model by adhering to scripting during patient encounters.

Table 1. Key Coordinated-Transitional Care (C-TraC) nurse role adaptations to create Resident-Coordinated Transitional Care (RC-TraC) resident role.

Area of adaptation	C-TraC nurse role	RC-TraC resident role
Patient populations[a]	Patients with nonresident primary care providers	Patients with resident primary care providers
Supervision requirements	Independently creates list of "red flags," triages patient concerns, and arranges clinic visit with primary care provider as needed	Requires RN C-TraC and attending physician oversight to create "red flags," triage patient concerns, and schedule clinic visits
	Must consult with primary care physician when new orders needed	Can provide new orders when indicated and notifies primary provider
Postdischarge patient contact	Telephonic contact only	May also see patients in clinic when indicated
Duration of role	Works full time in C-TraC role and follows all patients for the duration of program enrollment	Shares role with other resident physician colleagues; hands off patients to incoming resident after 4 weeks

a. C-TraC and RC-TraC function concurrently in a single VA hospital setting. RC-TraC enrolls only hospitalized patients who have internal medicine residents as primary care providers, whereas C-TraC enrolls only those who do not have internal medicine residents as primary care providers.

Resident and patient volumes

Between July 1, 2010 and June 30, 2013, RC-TraC residents cared for 721 patients, each resident following an average of 10.6 people during the rotation. Thirty-one residents completed at least one rotation during this period, representing 100% of residents with VA primary care clinics. Seventy-one resident RC-TraC rotations took place, or 2.3 per trainee. Fifty-six residents, all with university-affiliated clinics, did not experience RC-TraC.

Survey responses

The survey response rate was 95% (29 of 31 RC-TraC participants and 54 of 56 nonparticipants). RC-TraC participants were more likely to identify formal transitional care education experiences ($n = 28$, 97%) compared to nonparticipants ($n = 13$, 24%; $p < .001$).

Sustainability

The rotation continues in operation to this day and has been deemed to meet ACGME requirements for transitional care education by the residency program director. Rotation implementation did not require additional supervising physician or ancillary staff positions (Figure 1).

Discussion

RC-TraC successfully adapted the C-TraC nurse role for resident education, providing unique learning opportunities while still adhering to supervision requirements for trainees and basic tenets of transitional care for patients. Minimal changes were needed to incorporate a resident learner into the C-TraC RN role, and because it evolved from an existing rotation, it has not required additional staff full time equivalents to function, making it a low-cost intervention to implement. RC-TraC has been embraced as a sustainable, feasible program as a result, and the program director has deemed it to meet ACGME requirements for transitional care education. Further, because it exists concurrently with an active and successful C-TraC program, RC-TraC was well-accepted by Veterans and physician providers as a means of ensuring safe transitions and is well integrated into current hospital and clinic practices.

Through RC-TraC, residents witness the spectrum of illness and recovery frequently confronted by elderly patients with complex medical issues but rarely seen directly by the physician. Typical hospital ward experiences with these patients lack an outpatient follow-up component, and outpatient experiences miss the evolution of patients' recoveries between discharge and clinic visits. RC-TraC, however, places the resident at the forefront of the patient experience passing through this continuum of care, providing direct exposure to discharge process problems that cause readmissions.

As the survey results demonstrate, the majority of RC-TraC nonparticipants identified a transitional care as a gap in their training. RC-TraC residents, who consistently recognized their transitional care educational experience, could have greater insight into the challenges facing recently discharged patients. This may translate into better discharge practices and outpatient care of the recently discharged.

Unlike the majority of other resident-specific transitional care educational experiences, which are didactic based, RC-TraC provides a hands-on experience with care transitions (Buchanan & Besdine, 2011). RC-TraC affords opportunities to apply knowledge of best practices for discharge processes to actual patient care. Residents also witness instances where discharge planning fails to meet patients' needs and then work to resolve problems and avoid readmissions. This method of education, a combination of didactic and interactive learning, is regarded as most effective in altering physician behavior and could affect patient outcomes (Forsetlund et al., 2009).

RC-TraC could serve as a model for geriatric-based resident transitional care education at other sites and could be further adapted for other disciplines. C-TraC, upon which RC-TraC is based, has been disseminated to other VA and non-VA settings since inception, and RC-TraC may be similarly adaptable. RC-TraC's development could also serve as a model for creation of transitional care educational programs for nonphysicians, because many disciplines touch a patient during the discharge process. The iterative processes used to develop RC-TraC could account for differing educational backgrounds and supervision needs among other health care professional trainees.

The data presented here have limitations, primarily because launch of RC-TraC and its evaluation were conducted as pilot for feasibility and initial proof of concept. It is unclear whether RC-TraC has altered residents' discharge practices and improved care transitions. Whether RC-TraC is as effective as C-TraC in reducing readmissions is also unclear. Going forward, rigorous analysis of these endpoints is needed to better understand RC-TraC's impact, dissemination potential, and sustainability.

RC-TraC has been successful in its aims thus far by providing a feasible, sustainable, practice-based method to meet the need for resident education in transitional care best practices critical for safe management of older, complex adults. With education budgets shrinking and readmission penalties rising, a low-cost educational program such as RC-TraC is a promising option for transitional care education.

Acknowledgments

The authors would like to thank Michael Peregrim, MD, Laury L. Jensen, BSN, RN, Holly Isenhower Bottoms, MD, PharmD, and Mary K. Thompson, PhD for their contributions to the study concept and design. Also, thanks to Emily Schmitz, Michael Gehring, and Jacquelyn Mirr for their assistance with formatting the manuscript.

Funding

This work was supported by a VA Transformation-21 Grant (Patient-Centric Alternatives to Institutional Extended Care, PI: Kind) and the Madison VA Geriatrics Research, Education and Clinical Center (GRECC-Manuscript #2016-XX). Dr. Kind is also supported by a National Institute on Aging Beeson Career Development Award (K23AG034551 [PI: Kind], National Institute on Aging, The American Federation for Aging Research, The John A. Hartford Foundation, The Atlantic Philanthropies and The Starr Foundation). Additional support was provided by the University of Wisconsin School of Medicine and Public Health's Department of Medicine, and the Community-Academic Partnerships core of the University of Wisconsin Institute for Clinical and Translational Research (UW ICTR), grant 1UL1RR025011 from the Clinical and Translational Science Award (CTSA) program of the National Center for Research Resources, National Institutes of Health. No funding source had a role in the design and conduct of the study; collection, management, analysis, and interpretation of the data; or preparation, review, or approval of the manuscript, and decision to submit the manuscript for publication.

References

Accreditation Council for Graduate Medical Education. (2015). VI.B. Transitions of care. *ACGME program requirements for graduate medical education in internal medicine*. Retrieved from https://www.acgme.org/Portals/0/PFAssets/ProgramRequirements/140_internal_medicine_07012015.pdf

Buchanan, I. M., & Besdine, R. W. (2011). A systematic review of curricular interventions teaching transitional care to physicians-in-training and physicians. *Academic Medicine, 86*, 628–639. doi:10.1097/ACM.0b013e318212e36c

Callahan, C. M., Arling, G., Tu, W., Rosenman, M. B., Counsell, S. R., Stump, T. E., & Hendrie, H. C. (2012). Transitions in care among older adults with and without dementia. *Journal of the American Geriatrics Society, 60*(5), 813–820.

Coleman, E. A. (2003). Falling through the cracks: Challenges and opportunities for improving transitional care for persons with continuous complex care needs. *Journal of the American Geriatrics Society, 51*, 549–555. doi:10.1046/j.1532-5415.2003.51185.x

Coleman, E. A., Berenson, R. A. (2004). Lost in transition: Challenges and opportunities for improving the quality of transitional care. *Annals of Internal Medicine, 141*, 533–536.

Coleman, E. A., & Chalmers, S. (2006). The care transitions intervention: Results of a randomized controlled trial. *Archives of Internal Medicine, 166*, 1822–1828

Coleman, E. A., Min, S., Chomiak, A., & Kramer, A. M. (2004). Posthospital care transitions: Patterns, complications, and risk identification. *HSR: Health Services Research, 39*(5), 1449–1466.

Coleman, E. A., Parry, C., Chalmers, S., & Min, S. (2006). The care transitions intervention: Results of a randomized controlled trial. *Archives of Internal Medicine, 166*, 1822–1828. doi:10.1001/archinte.166.17.1822

Coleman, E. A., Smith, J. D., Frank, J. C., Eilertsen, T. B., Thiare, J. N., & Kramer, A. N. (2002). Development and testing of a measure designed to assess the quality of care transitions. *International Journal of Integrated Care, 2*, Epub.

Coleman, E. A., Smith, J. D., Raha, D., & Min, S. (2005). Posthospital medication discrepancies: Prevalance and contributing factors. *Archives of Internal Medicine, 165*, 1842–1847. doi:10.1001/archinte.165.16.1842

Forsetlund, L., Bjorndal, A., Rashidian, A., Jamtvedt, G., O'Brien, M. A., Wolf, F. M. . . . Oxman, A. D. (2009). Continuing education meetings and workshops: Effects on professional practice and health care outcomes. *Cochrane Database Systematic Reviews, 2*, CD003030. doi:10.1002/14651858.CD003030.pub2

Forster, A. J., Murff, H. J., Peterson, J. F., Gandhi, T. K., Bates, D. W. (2003). The incidence and severity of adverse events affecting patients after discharge from the hospital. *Annals of Internal Medicine, 138*(3), 161–167.

Fuji, K. T., Abbott, A. A., & Norris, J. F. (2013). Exploring care transitions from patient, caregiver, and health-care provider perspectives. *Clinical Nursing Research, 22*(3), 258–274.

Gerteis, J., Izrael, D., Deitz, D., LeRoy, L., Ricciardi, R., Miller, T., & Basu, J. (2014). *Multiple chronic conditions chartbook* (AHRQ Publications, No. Q14-0038). Rockville, MD: Agency for Healthcare Research and Quality. Retrieved from.

Hirschman, K., Shaid, E., McCauley, K., Pauly, M., & Naylor, M. (2015). Continuity of Care: The transitional care model. *OJIN: The Online Journal of Issues in Nursing, 20*(3), 1.

James, J. (2013). *Medicare Hospital Readmissions Reduction Program* (Health Affairs/RWJF Health Policy Brief). Retrieved from: http://www.rwjf.org/content/dam/farm/reports/issue_briefs/2013/rwjf408708

Jencks, S. F., Williams, M. V., Coleman, E. A. (2009). Rehospitalizations among patients in the Medicare fee-for-service program. *New England Journal of Medicine, 360*(14), 1418–1428.

Kind A. J. H. (2012). *The Department of Veterans Affairs Coordinated-Transitional Care (C-TraC) Program Toolkit*. Madison, WI: Madison VA Geriatric Research and Clinical Centers (GRECC) and the UW Health Innovation Program. Retrieved from: http://www.hipxchange.org/C-TraC.

Kind, A. J. H., Jensen, L., Barczi, S., Bridges, A., Kordahl, R., Smith, M. A., & Asthana, S. (2012). Low-cost transitional care with nurse managers making mostly phone contact with patients cut rehospitalization at a VA hospital. *Health Affairs (Millwood)*, 31, 2659–2668. doi:10.1377/hlthaff.2012.0366

King, B. D., Gilmore-Bykovskyi, A., Roiland, R., Polnaszek, B. E., Bowers, B. J., & Kind, A. J. (2013). The consequences of poor communication during transitions from hospital to skilled nursing facility: A qualitative study. *Journal of the American Geriatrics Society*, 61(7), 1095–1102.

Moore, C., Wisnivesky, J., Williams, S., & McGinn, T. (2003). Medical errors related to discontinuity of care from an inpatient to an outpatient setting. *Journal of General Internal Medicine*, 18, 646–651.

Patient Protection and Affordable Care Act, H.R. 3590, Sec. 3025 (2010).

Riebschleger, M., & Philibert, I. (2011). New standards for transitions of care: Discussion and justification. In I. Philibert & S. Amis (Eds.), *The ACGME 2011 duty hour standards: Enhancing quality of care, supervision, and resident professional development* (pp. 57–59). Chicago, IL: Accreditation Council for Graduate Medical Education.

Appendix

Resident-Coordinated Transitional Care (RC-TraC) curriculum elements

Curriculum topics	Main point(s) covered	Exemplar references used to inform curriculum content
Scope of hospital readmission problem[a,b]	Rehospitalizations are common among Medicare beneficiaries Rehospitalizations are costly Rehospitalizations often occur before scheduled clinic follow-up Many rehospitalizations are preventable	Jencks, Williams, & Coleman (2009)
Factors that contribute to preventable hospital readmissions and individual risk for experiencing readmission[a,b,c,d]	Factors that contribute to preventable readmission: Poor communication between care settings and provider teams Inadequate patient/caregiver education in self-management Limited clinician training in transitional care Individual risk factors for experiencing readmission: Difficulty accessing needed services Cognitive impairment Difficulty with activities of daily living Depression Discharge to a skilled nursing facility Substance abuse disorders History of previous hospitalization Unrecognized language, health literacy and cultural differences between providers and patients	Callahan et al. (2012) Coleman (2003) Jencks, Williams, & Coleman (2009)
Impact of poor transitional care[a,b,d]	Impact on patients/caregivers: Preventable medication errors and other adverse events often occur Follow-up of important issues may be delayed or missed Increased patient and caregiver dissatisfaction and stress Complicated transitions often necessitate increased contact with medical system. Impact on health care systems: Increased stress among staff accepting patients from acute care to skilled nursing facilities. Delays in care caused by inadequate transitional care practices in the acute care setting reflect poorly on skilled nursing facilities receiving discharged patients Hospitals with disproportionately high readmission rates face reimbursement penalties	Coleman, Smith, Raha, & Min (2005) Coleman (2003) Coleman & Berenson (2004) Forster, Murff, Peterson, Gandhi, & Bates (2003) Fuji, Abbott, & Norris (2013) King et al. (2013) Moore, Wisnivesky, Williams, & McGinn (2003) Patient Protection and Affordable Care Act (2010) James (2013)

(Continued)

(Continued).

Curriculum topics	Main point(s) covered	Exemplar references used to inform curriculum content
Best practices for transitional care (based on Coleman's Four Pillars)[a,b,d]	Components include: Timely transfer of critical information to the next care setting Individualization of care plans to meet each patient's needs and align with his or her goals and preferences. Preparation of the patient/caregiver for care at next location, including setting expectations and making explicit follow-up plans Education and empowerment regarding self-management, including monitoring for key symptoms, medication reconciliation and teaching, and contact information for obtaining assistance when concerns arise	Coleman et al. (2002) Coleman (2003) Coleman & Chalmers (2006)
Health Policy measures targeting care transitions[a,b]	Hospitals are penalized when rates of unplanned readmissions exceed standards. New billing codes increase reimbursement for post-discharge care coordination.	Patient Protection and Affordable Care Act (2010). James (2013)
RC-TraC Model and Protocols[a,b,d]	Shared goals of C-TraC and RC-TraC: Educate/empower patient in medication management Ensure appropriate medical follow-up Educate patient regarding "red flag" symptoms Ensure patient knows who to contact with questions RC-Trac protocol elements: In-hospital meeting before discharge Rapid and regular telephone follow-up with medication review and review of "red flags"	Kind (2012) Kind et al. (2012)

a. Covered in assigned reading (occupies 2–3 hours of total rotation time).
b. Covered in narrated presentation (occupies 1 hour of total rotation time).
c. Covered in online learning modules (occupies 3–4 hours of total rotation time).
d. Covered in experiential learning (occupies 80–90 hours of total rotation time, including in-person meetings, telephone contacts, and clinic visits).

Geriatrics fellowship training and the role of geriatricians in older adult cancer care: A survey of geriatrics fellowship directors

Ronald J. Maggiore ⓘ, Kathryn E. Callahan, Janet A. Tooze, Ira R. Parker, Tina Hsu, and Heidi D. Klepin

ABSTRACT

The number of older adults with cancer is growing, necessitating more collaborative training in geriatric principles and cancer care. The authors administered a web-based survey to U.S. geriatrics program directors (PDs) addressing cancer-specific training and perspectives on optimal training content and roles for geriatricians in cancer care. Of 140 PDs contacted, 67 (48%) responded. Topics considered very important in training included cancer screening (79%) and cancer-related pain management (70%). Respondents strongly agreed that some of the geriatrician's roles in cancer care included assessing functional status (64%) and assessing physical/cognitive function for goals of care (64%). About one half (54%) agreed that having a standardized geriatric oncology curriculum overall was important. The presence of a geriatric oncologist, requiring cancer-based rotations, being affiliated with a cancer center, or being internal versus family medicine-based did not affect this response. Despite this high level of support, cancer-related skills and knowledge warrant better definition and integration into current geriatrics training. This survey establishes potential areas for future educational collaborations between geriatrics and oncology training programs.

Introduction

By 2030, approximately two thirds of patients with cancer will be age 65 years and older (American Society of Clinical Oncology, 2014; Smith et al., 2009). Therefore, physicians will need training in how best to manage the increasing number of older adults with cancer (OACs) and aging-related risks such as frailty and multimorbidity. Only 47% of hematology/oncology trainees in the United States report receiving at least one dedicated lecture on caring for OACs (Maggiore et al., 2014). In the United Kingdom, 66% reported no formal geriatric oncology training (Kalsi et al., 2013). In a survey of U.S. hematology/oncology fellowship program directors (PDs), 32% reported having a formal curriculum including geriatric oncology (Naeim et al., 2010). Nonetheless, most hematology/oncology trainees and PDs value geriatric oncology training (Maggiore et al., 2014; Naeim et al., 2010). Although these oncology fellowship-based studies provide some insight into the training knowledge gaps in the care of OACs, little is known about such training needs from geriatrics fellowship perspective. Ultimately, optimal health care delivery models for OACs will require collaborations between oncology and geriatrics, beginning with fellowship training.

Cancer is one of several comorbidities for which geriatrics fellows must demonstrate knowledge, but cancer care is not a mandatory component of their training, according to the Accreditation Council for Graduate Medical Education (ACGME; 2016). Approaches to integrating cancer care into geriatrics training programs may vary widely, thereby warranting further investigation into the current training environment. We performed a survey-based study of geriatrics PDs to query them about their (1) current geriatrics fellowship training landscape related to the care of OACs, (2) perceptions of optimal roles for geriatricians in caring for OACs, and (3) attitudes about geriatrics fellowship training content related to the care of OACs. We also looked at whether various program factors were associated with the endorsement of a geriatric oncology curriculum.

Method

Participants

Potential participants were PDs or associate PDs from ACGME-accredited U.S. geriatrics fellowship programs.

Measures

A modified Delphi process among a panel of U.S. geriatric oncologists affiliated with the Cancer and Aging Research Group (geriatricians, oncologists, and allied health professionals interested in geriatric oncology research) developed the survey items. Three rounds of reviews led to a consensus. The survey consisted of six sections (Appendix): (1) demographics including years as program director (Part A); (2) didactic and clinical experiences offered regarding care of OACs (Parts B and C); (3) attitudes toward geriatric oncology principles in geriatrics fellowship training (Parts D and E); and (4) perceptions of geriatricians' roles in caring for OACs (Part F). A section for open-ended comments was provided.

Procedures

The American Geriatrics Society's (AGS) Fellowship Directors' Committee provided email addresses of PDs/associate PDs of ACGME-accredited U.S. geriatrics fellowship programs ($N = 140$ of 152 accredited programs). The survey was administered using Research Electronic Data Capture (REDCap^M) software (Harris et al., 2009). Institutional Review Board approval was obtained with a waiver of written consent.

PDs received a short description of the study's purpose and were assumed to provide consent if they answered the survey. Potential respondents received the survey link by e-mail, and two reminders, between May and December 2014.

Analysis

Responses were collectively organized by emerging themes rather than based on survey section. Data are presented as frequencies and percentages based on all responses, unless otherwise noted. Chi-square tests were utilized to compare whether an endorsement of a standard curriculum varied by four characteristics: presence of geriatric oncologist expert, mandatory geriatric oncology training experiences/rotations, cancer center affiliation, or program based in internal medicine versus family medicine. A two-sided alpha level of 0.05 was the threshold for statistical significance. Data were analyzed using SAS software (v 9.4).

Results

Sixty-seven of the 140 potential respondents (48%) provided at least one response in all survey sections. Although e-mail addresses were not linked to these responses, the survey software allowed respondents to be tracked; as a result, these 67 respondents were from unique programs. Respondents were experienced PDs (about one half with ≥ 6 years) and were mostly at academically oriented, internal medicine–based geriatrics fellowship programs with an affiliated cancer center (Table 1). Ten percent offered formal geriatrics-medical oncology fellowship training. Furthermore, 62% responded that collaborations between geriatrics and oncology divisions were "highly likely" or "likely" to support a geriatrics fellow interested in geriatric oncology.

Three emergent themes arose within the responses for purposes of conceptually organizing and reporting the study data:

Current geriatrics fellowship training landscape related to the care of OACs

Most PDs reported having formal teaching addressing care of OACs, usually in lectures or seminars (81%). Other methods included readings or journal clubs (75%); case studies or conferences (55%); workshops (6%); and geriatric oncology modules from the American Society of Clinical Oncology (ASCO) (1%). About 30% of programs dedicated 4 to 7 hours of instruction, whereas 46% dedicated 1 to 3 hours to teaching cancer care. Only 39% reported mandatory clinical experiences in cancer care for older adults, whereas 46% reported offering clinical electives in geriatric oncology. The time dedicated to clinical experiences in caring for OACs and formal teaching of geriatric oncology topics varied (Table 1). Several respondents reported in free-text comments that palliative medicine rotations were an opportunity for fellows to learn more about caring for OACs.

Perceptions of optimal roles for geriatricians caring for OACs

The majority of respondents reported that geriatricians in general should serve in consultative as well as primary-care roles (92%), rather than as consultants alone (8%). Among free-text comments obtained, a few PDs pointed out the importance of geriatricians' playing a role in primary palliative care ($n = 2$), transitions of care including end-of-life care ($n = 2$), primary care for OACs with dementia ($n = 1$), and equal comanagement of OACs throughout the cancer trajectory alongside the oncologist ($n = 5$). More specifically, many PDs strongly agreed that optimal roles for geriatricians in care for OACs include (1) determining functional status, as a consultant; (2) determining physical/cognitive status in context of goals of care; and (3) participating in cancer care decision making when the geriatrician is the primary care provider (Table 2). Respondents felt geriatricians should assume more of a primary care provider role during active cancer therapy (67%), at completion of cancer therapy (79%), and when the patient is cancer free for at least 5 years

Table 1. Characteristics of survey respondents and representative programs ($N = 67$).

Characteristic	n (%)
Years as program director/associate program director	
0–1 year	9 (13)
2 years	9 (13)
3–5 years	15 (22)
6–10 years	22 (33)
> 10 years	12 (18)
Sponsoring department for geriatrics fellowship	
Internal medicine	45 (67)
Family medicine	21 (31)
Both	1 (1)
Length of Geriatrics Fellowship Program(s) offered	
1 year	63 (94)
2 years	21 (31)
2 years with option of additional research years	8 (12)
Number of fellowship positions per year[a]	
1–2	28 (44)
3	12 (19)
4	16 (25)
≥ 5	8 (13)
Formal geriatric oncology fellowship training pathway available	7 (10)
Affiliated with a cancer center or cancer program with clinical component	63 (95)
Fellowship program likely or highly likely to collaborate with cancer center [b,c]	38 (62)
Presence of oncologist with expertise in geriatric oncology[b, < d]	24 (39)
If present, does he/she provide education for geriatric fellows[e]	14 (58)
If not present, who provides geriatric oncology education[f]	22 (58)
Geriatric faculty	10 (26)
No individual provides this content	6 (16)
Other	
Didactic time dedicated to the care of OAC[g,]	
0	6 (9)
< 1 hour	4 (6)
1–3 hours	31 (46)
4–7 hours	21 (31)
> 7 hours	5 (7)
Clinical experience time dedicated to the care of OAC	
< 2 hours	19 (29)
2–4 hours	8 (12)
5–12 hours	11 (17)
13–20 hours	15 (23)
> 20 hours	12 (18)

Note. OAC = Older adults with cancer
a. $n = 64$; 3 participants missing
b. Among participants with a cancer center or cancer program with clinical component, $N = 63$
c. $n = 61$; 2 participants missing
d. $n = 62$; 1 participant missing
e. Among participants with oncologist with expertise in geriatric oncology at cancer center, $n = 24$
f. Among participants without oncologist with expertise in geriatric oncology at cancer center, $n = 38$
g. $n = 65$; 2 participants missing

(89%). However, only 57% of respondents strongly agreed or agreed that geriatricians' roles included overseeing cancer surveillance and managing late-term effects of cancer therapy. Nearly all respondents thought geriatricians should be primary care providers and consultants in caring for OACs, not just consultants (92% vs. 8%).

Attitudes about geriatrics fellowship training content related to the care of OACs

Most respondents agreed that geriatric oncology principles should be integrated in geriatrics fellowship training through a standardized curriculum (Table 2). Respondents' attitudes toward a standardized geriatric oncology curriculum did not differ across programs based on presence of a geriatric oncologist expert (66.7% "yes" vs. 47.4% "no/don't know", $p = .14$), mandatory formal geriatric oncology training experiences/rotations (60.0% "yes" vs. 52.5%

Table 2. Agreement with statements regarding geriatric oncology content and roles for geriatricians in the care of the older adult with cancer.

Item	N	Strongly agree	Agree	% Neutral	Disagree	Strongly disagree
Geriatrics fellowship curriculum should:						
Include geriatric oncology components	66	26	51	15	6	1
Be standardized to meet geriatrics fellow training needs	66	21	33	29	15	2
Geriatrician's role in the care of the older adult with cancer:						
Determining functional status as consultant	66	64	33	3	0	0
Determining physical and cognitive status in context of goals of care at the time of diagnosis	64	64	33	3	0	0
Participating in cancer care decision making when geriatrician is the primary care provider	66	58	33	6	3	0
Participating in developing a patient's cancer survivorship plan with the oncologist	66	33	53	14	0	0
Being solely responsible for a patient's primary care management during active cancer therapy	66	20	47	18	14	1
Being solely responsible for a patient's primary care management upon completion of cancer therapy	66	32	47	14	8	0
Being solely responsible for a patient's primary care when cancer-free for ≥ 5 years	65	34	55	6	5	0
Being responsible for cancer-specific surveillance/ monitoring of late-term cancer therapy-related adverse effects when cancer-free ≥ 5 years	65	22	35	26	17	0

Table 3. Endorsed importance of geriatric oncology content.

Item	N	Very important	Important	% Neutral	Somewhat important	Not important
Cancer screening in older adults	66	79	18	3	0	0
Assess and manage cancer-related pain	66	70	24	3	1	1
Assess and optimize functional status in vulnerable older adults throughout cancer trajectory	65	65	32	3	0	0
Assess cognitive status in cancer care decision making	65	65	28	8	0	0
Assess geriatric syndromes in cancer therapy decision making	65	62	32	6	0	0
Assess geriatric syndromes in supportive care decision making	65	58	34	8	0	0
Assess and optimize functional status in fit patients throughout cancer trajectory	66	55	33	9	3	0
Assess and manage psychological issues throughout cancer trajectory	64	53	41	6	0	0
Assess and manage comorbidities	66	53	41	5	1	0
Assess and manage cancer therapy-related adverse events	64	41	42	11	5	1
Broadly understand cancer therapies for most common cancers in older adults	66	26	56	12	3	3
Utilize cancer-focused comprehensive geriatric assessment instruments	66	17	52	24	6	1

"no", $p = .55$), cancer center affiliation (56.5% "yes" vs. 57.5% "no", $p = .94$), or internal medicine versus family medicine (54.5% "internal" vs. 52.4% "family," $p = .87$).Most respondents felt that screening and assessment skills for care of OACs were "very important" for fellows to learn (Table 3). Few PDs defined these areas in care of OACs as very important: assessing and managing cancer therapy-related adverse events, broadly understanding therapies for prevalent cancers in OACs, and utilizing cancer-focused geriatric assessment items.

Discussion

Most respondents believe that cancer care and geriatric oncology principles are relevant to their trainees. However, formal didactic teaching or clinical experiences on this topic, though prevalent in our sample, vary widely. Many respondents stated they would support a standardized geriatric oncology curriculum, and such efforts have been reported (Eid et al., 2015). This survey's results identified areas that geriatrics fellowship PDs identified as important for future geriatricians and their roles in care for OACs. These can be the foundation for collaborations between geriatrics and oncology educators, to determine common core competencies to benefit trainees from both fields, particularly because most of the programs reported being affiliated with a cancer center.

General challenges to collaborations between geriatrics and oncology fellowship programs include difficulties in scheduling clinical and didactic experiences, differences in training requirements, and the lack of formally accredited combined fellowship programs. These issues may partly explain underuse of extramural resources, such as ASCO's online geriatric oncology modules. Such modules could provide didactic support for programs with more limited access to faculty or a cancer center.

This study highlights educational content and roles that geriatricians perceive as most important to support their care of OACs. This information is critical to designing education to support effective models of care. Respondents identified application of geriatric assessment findings (i.e., cognitive and functional status) and formulation of goals of care as key skills for optimal care of OACs. These areas of content overlap with unmet training needs in oncology fellowships. Hematology/oncology fellows in the United Kingdom identified geriatric assessment skills and recognizing geriatric syndromes that affect cancer therapy decision making as areas where they needed improved training (Kalsi et al., 2013; Maggiore et al., 2014). These fellows receive less formal training in observation/feedback of functional assessment of OACs or end-of-life care discussions versus procedure-based, "traditional" oncology skills (e.g., bone marrow biopsies) (Buss et al., 2011; Maggiore et al., 2014).

Combined geriatrics and hematology/oncology training may allow geriatrics and hematology/oncology fellows to better learn from one another. For example, incorporating cognitive and functional assessments into care of OACs can be an opportunity for integrated, milestone-oriented training for geriatrics and hematology/oncology fellows, incorporated into ACGME-required training now in place. Other interdisciplinary care venues can foster improved training for geriatrics and cancer trainees (Akthar et al., 2017). For example, tumor board conferences allow geriatricians and oncologists to collaborate and thereby influence shared cancer treatment decision making for OACs (Blanc et al., 2014).

Many patients who use palliative medicine services are OACs. Because geriatrics and medical oncology fellows must rotate through and attain competencies in palliative medicine, it may be a natural place to integrate geriatric oncology education. However, it is unclear to what extent geriatric oncology is covered during the palliative medicine experiences of geriatrics fellows, which can be affected by availability of resources (e.g., type of clinical setting) and other factors (Cao et al., 2015).

There was less consensus regarding the geriatrician's role in managing cancer therapy-related adverse events or focusing curricular content on specific cancer therapies. Given the time constraints (usually 1 year of training) and specific requirements of geriatrics fellowship programs, there is likely little flexibility to add more cancer-based didactics or clinical experiences for these topics to be addressed. Alternatively, a comanagement model may be more preferred by geriatricians in that some or all of these knowledge and skill-sets be delegated to the hematologist or oncologist specifically. This framework allows the geriatrician to focus more on "gero-centric" issues across the cancer care continuum, such as functional and cognitive issues to which the survey results appear to allude. Taken together, these data provide a framework for future collaborations between geriatrics and oncology educators to determine common core competencies for trainees.

The current study has limitations. The AGS fellowship directors' committee list is representative of, but not entirely inclusive of, all active programs, and the contribution of program and program directors' information is entirely voluntary. Not all intended recipients completed the survey, despite reminders. The most important limitation is potential response bias in interpreting survey results. The program directors who responded might inherently be more supportive of geriatric oncology education. To examine potential response bias, we used late responders (i.e., last quartile to complete) as a proxy for non-responders, a technique used in other studies (Kellerman & Herold, 2001), and compared them to the first quartile of respondents. Early and late survey responders did not significantly differ in ratings of importance of screening and assessment skills for care of OACs (data not shown). This lack of difference suggests that nonresponders' attitudes may not differ from survey responders. Importantly, our response rate is comparable to that in other survey-based studies; physician surveys have an average response rate of 54% (Asch, Jedrziewski, & Christakis, 1997), though specialist responses may be as low as 27% (Cunningham et al., 2015). Furthermore, non-response bias may not be as meaningful in physician surveys, based on the lack of significant differences between responders and non-responders in studies exploring this issue (Draugalis, Coons, & Plaza, 2008; Kellerman & Herold, 2001).

This is the first study to evaluate geriatrics fellowship program directors' views on the current training landscape for geriatrics fellows regarding care of OACs, perceptions of geriatricians' roles in such care, and their attitudes toward the training needs for delivery of such care. In this survey of geriatrics fellowship program directors, geriatric oncology principles were considered important for geriatrics fellows to learn. The new information gained from this study provides a foundation for educational programming that best meets the needs of future OAC care-providers. Future studies are required to develop a formal needs assessment for OAC care for geriatrics fellows. Furthermore, strategies in creating opportunities for collaborative education in geriatrics and hematology/oncology will continue to be needed.

Conclusion

Types of didactic and clinical resources for geriatrics fellows vary across programs regarding OAC care. Most respondents felt that geriatricians can serve specific roles within this context. Further studies are needed to determine consensus regarding (1) a geriatric oncology curriculum and (2) augmented educational resources relevant for trainees caring for OACs in their careers.

Acknowledgments

We thank Erin Obrusniak and members of the American Geriatrics Society for facilitating the development and conduct of this study. We also thank Karen Klein in the Wake Forest Clinical and Translational Science Institute (which is supported by UL1 TR001420; Principal Investigator: King Li) for reviewing and editing the manuscript. An abstract of this study was accepted and presented at the Annual Meeting of the American Geriatrics Society on 15 May 2015.

Conflicts of interest

The authors declare no conflicts of interest (disclosures table below). The authors affirm that this manuscript has not previously been published, nor has it simultaneously been submitted for review for publication at another journal.

Funding

This research was supported by the Biostatistics and Bioinformatics Shared Resource of the Comprehensive Cancer Center of Wake Forest University (P30 CA012197, Principal Investigator: Boris Pasche).

ORCID

Ronald J. Maggiore ⬤ http://orcid.org/0000-0002-2445-7481

References

Accreditation Council for Graduate Medical Education. (2016, February 8). *Program requirements for graduate medical education in geriatric medicine (family medicine or internal medicine).* Retrieved from https://www.acgme.org/acgmeweb/Portals/0/PFAssets/ProgramRequirements/125-151_geriatric_medicine_2016_1-YR.pdf

Akthar, A. S., Ganai, S., Hahn, O. M., Maggiore, R. J., Cohen, E. E. W., Posner, M., ... Golden, D. W. (2017). Interdisciplinary oncology education: A national survey of trainees and program directors in the United States. *Journal of Cancer Education*, Advance online publication.

American Society of Clinical Oncology. (2014, March 10). *The state of cancer in America, 2014.* Retrieved from http://www.asco.org/practice-research/cancer-care-america.

Asch, D. A., Jedrziewski, M. K., & Christakis, N. A. (1997). Response rates to mail surveys published in medical journals. *Journal of Clinical Epidemiology*, 50(10), 1129–1136. doi:10.1016/S0895-4356(97)00126-1

Blanc, M., Dialla, O., Manckoundia, P., Arveux, P., Dabakuyo, S., & Quipourt, V. (2014). Influence of the geriatric oncology consultation on the final therapeutic decision in elderly subjects with cancer: Analysis of 191 patients. *Journal of Nutrition, Health, and Aging*, 18(1), 76–82. doi:10.1007/s12603-013-0377-0

Buss, M. K., Lessens, D. K., Sullivan, A. M., Von Roenn, J., Arnold, R. M., & Block, S. D. (2011). Hematology/oncology fellows' training in palliative care: Results of a national survey. *Cancer*, 117(18), 4304–4311. doi:10.1002/cncr.25952

Cao, Q., Lee, T. J., Hayes, S. M., Nye, A. M., Hamrick, I., Patil, S., & Steinweg, K. K. (2015). Are geriatric medicine fellows prepared for the important skills of hospice and palliative care? *American Journal of Hospice and Palliative Care, 32*, 322–328. doi:10.1177/1049909113517050

Cunningham, C. T., Quan, H., Hemmelgarn, B., Noseworthy, T., Beck, C. A., Dixon, E., . . . Jetté, N. (2015). Exploring physician specialist response rates to web-based surveys. *BioMed Central Medical Research Methodology, 15*(32), 1–8. doi:10.1186/s12874-015-0016-z

Draugalis, J. R., Coons, S. J., & Plaza, C. M. (2008). Best practices for survey research reports: A synopsis for authors and reviewers. *American Journal of Pharmaceutical Education, 72*(1), 11. doi:10.5688/aj720111

Eid, A., Hughes, C., Karuturi, M., Reyes, C., Yorio, J., & Holmes, H. (2015). An interprofessionally developed geriatric oncology curriculum for hematology-oncology fellows. *Journal of Geriatric Oncology, 6*(2), 165–173. doi:10.1016/j.jgo.2014.11.003

Harris, P. A., Taylor, R., Thielke, R., Payne, J., Gonzalez, N., & Conde, J. G. (2009). Research electronic data capture (REDCap^{TM}) - A metadata-driven methodology and workflow process for providing translational research informatics support. *Journal of Biomedical Informatics, 42*(2), 377–381. doi:10.1016/j.jbi.2008.08.010

Kalsi, T., Payne, S., Brodie, H., Mansi, J., Wang, Y., & Harari, D. (2013). Are the UK oncology trainees adequately informed about the needs of older people with cancer? *British Journal of Cancer, 108*, 1936–1941. doi:10.1038/bjc.2013.204

Kellerman, S. E., & Herold, J. (2001). Physician responses to surveys. *American Journal of Preventive Medicine, 20*(1), 61–67. doi:10.1016/S0749-3797(00)00258-0

Maggiore, R. J., Dale, W., Buss, M. K., Hurria, A., Chapman, A. E., Dotan, E., . . . Mohile, S. G. (2014). Survey of geriatric oncology (geri onc) training among hematology/oncology (hem/onc) fellows. *Journal of Clinical Oncology, 32*, (Suppl), abstr e20519.

Naeim, A., Hurria, A., Rao, A., Cohen, H., Heflin, M., & Seo, P. (2010). The need for an aging and cancer curriculum for hematology/oncology trainees. *Journal of Geriatric Oncology, 1*(2), 109–113. doi:10.1016/j.jgo.2010.08.004

Smith, B. D., Smith, G. L., Hurria, A., Hortobagyi, G. N., & Buchholz, T. A. (2009). Future of cancer incidence in the United States: Burdens upon an aging, changing nation. *Journal of Clinical Oncology, 27*(17), 2758–2765. doi:10.1200/JCO.2008.20.8983

Appendix

Oncology Curricular Content of United States-Based Geriatric Medicine Fellowship Training Programs

This survey should take approximately 5–10 minutes to complete. You may save answers and return at a later time to complete the survey if needed. Your participation is appreciated.

A. Geriatric Medicine Fellowship Training Program Profile

A1. How many years have you served as your institution's Geriatric Medicine Fellowship Program's director?

Please Specify: _____ years

A2. Which department/division <u>sponsors</u> your Geriatric Medicine Fellowship Training Program?

□ Family Medicine

□ Internal Medicine

□ Other: (Please specify) _____

A3. What type(s) of geriatric medicine fellowship training does your institution offer? (Please select all answers that apply.)

□ 1-year fellowship

□ 2-year fellowship

□ Other: (Please Specify) _____

A4. How many geriatric medicine fellowship training slots (not including joint/integrated fellowships) are available <u>each year</u> at your institution?

Please specify: _____

A5. Does your institution offer a training pathway focusing upon <u>both</u> geriatric medicine and oncology fellowship training?
Yes → No
If yes, do you offer a combined fellowship for dual certification in geriatrics and oncology?
Yes → No
B. Geriatric Medicine Fellowship Training Program Oncology Curricular Content
The following questions are addressing training experiences of the geriatric medicine fellows in your program, excluding those fellows who are in a joint Geriatric Medicine/Oncology Program.
B1. Which of the following didactic approaches does your institution's Geriatric Medicine Fellowship Program utilize in teaching geriatric oncology to its fellows? (Please check all that apply.)
□ Readings/journal club
□ Lectures/seminars
□ Case studies or case conferences
□ Workshops
□ ASCO university online training modules
□ Other online training modules
□ Other: (Please Specify): _____
□ None of the above
B2. How many hours of didactic education (e.g. lecture, seminar, etc.), directly related to cancer in older adults, is provided to your geriatric medicine fellows <u>during their clinical training</u>?
□ None
□ < 1 hour
□ 1 – 3 hours
□ 4 – 7 hours
□ > 7 hours
B3. Does your geriatric medicine fellowship curriculum include one or more <u>mandatory</u> clinical training exposure(s)/experience(s) that is/are directly related to cancer in older adults?
Yes → No
If "Yes": Please describe.
B4. Does your geriatric medicine fellowship offer <u>elective/selective</u> clinical training experience(s) that is/are directly related to cancer in older adults?
Yes → No
If "Yes": Please describe.
B5. How many hours of <u>clinical</u> training exposure, directly related to cancer in older adults, are provided to your geriatric medicine fellows?
□ < 2 hours
□ 2 – 4 hours
□ 5 – 8 hours
□ 9 – 12 hours
□ 13 – 20 hours
□ >20 hours
C. Oncology Program Status at Your Institution
C1. Does your institution have a cancer center or cancer program that has a clinical care component?
Yes → No
If "No": Please proceed to Question C6.
C2. Does your institution's Cancer Center have a National Cancer Institute "Comprehensive Cancer Center" designation?
Yes → No Do Not Know
C3. How likely is it that your fellowship program could collaborate with your institution's cancer center/cancer program to accommodate a geriatric medicine fellow's interest in oncology?
□ Highly likely □ Likely □ Not sure □ Unlikely □ Highly unlikely
C4. Is there a faculty member at your institution's Cancer Center who has expertise focusing upon the delivery of cancer care to older adult patients?

Yes → No Do Not Know
If "No" or "Do Not Know" please proceed to Question C6.
C5. Does this faculty member provide Geriatric Oncology-focused instruction to your Geriatric Medicine fellows?
Yes → No
If "Yes": Please proceed to Section D.

	Strongly agree	Agree	Neutral	Disagree	Strongly disagree
D1. Geriatric medicine fellowship training programs should include dedicated curricular components focusing upon geriatric oncology.					
D2. A standard curriculum should be established targeting the geriatric oncology training needs of geriatric medicine fellows.					

C6. If your institution does not have an oncologist focused on cancer care in older persons, who provides this training to your fellows?
☐ No one. Geriatric oncology instruction/training is not provided.

	Very important	Important	Neutral	Somewhat important	Not important
E1. Screening for common cancers of older adults					
E2. Having a broad understanding of cancer therapies (e.g., curative vs. palliative intent, potential toxicities, goals of care) for treatment of common cancers in older adults (i.e., prostate, breast, colorectal, lung, lymphoma)					
E3. Assessing cognitive status within the framework of cancer care decision-making capacity					
E4. Assessing for geriatric syndromes that may potentially affect cancer therapy decision making					
E5. Assessing for geriatric syndromes that may potentially impact cancer supportive care decision making					
E6. Utilizing cancer-focused Comprehensive Geriatric Assessment instruments					
E7. Assessing and managing medical comorbidities throughout the patient's cancer care					
E8. Assessing and optimizing functional status in fit older adult patients throughout their cancer care trajectory					
E9. Assessing and optimizing functional status in vulnerable older adult patients throughout their cancer care trajectory					
E10. Assessing and managing cancer-related pain					
E11. Assessing and managing adverse effects/events related to cancer therapy					
E12. Assessing and managing psychological issues throughout the patient's cancer care trajectory					

☐ One or more of our geriatric medicine faculty.
☐ A noninstitution-affiliated oncologist with geriatric medicine expertise.
☐ Other
D. Oncology training in geriatrics fellowship
What is your level of agreement with regard to the following statements?
E. Curricular content regarding care of older patients in geriatrics training
How important is it to include the following topics in a Geriatric Medicine Fellowship Training curriculum?
E13. In your opinion, which other geriatric oncology-focused curricular topics should be included in a geriatric medicine fellowship training curriculum?

Please Specify: _____

E14. In your opinion, which of the following geriatric oncology-focused educational opportunities would benefit your geriatric medicine fellows? (Check all that apply)

□ Half-day symposium/workshop in conjunction with a national or regional conference
□ Full-day symposium/workshop in conjunction with a national or regional conference
□ Web-based training modules
□ Webinars
□ Other: (Please specify) _____
□ None of the above

E15. What percentage of your geriatric medicine fellows attend at least one American Geriatrics Society Annual Scientific meeting during her/his training?

□ 0% – 25%
□ 26% – 50%
□ 51% – 75%
□ 76% – 100%

	Strongly agree	Agree	Neutral	Disagree	Strongly disagree
F1. Determining a patient's functional status/"medical vulnerability" in a consultative role					
F2. Determining a patient's physical and cognitive function in relation to goals of care at the time of cancer diagnosis in a consultative role					
F3. Participating in the cancer care treatment decision-making process when the geriatrician is the physician of record of the cancer patient					
F4. Participating in the development of a survivorship care plan for older adults with cancer (in conjunction with the hematologist/oncologist)					
F5. Being solely responsible for the patient's primary care management during the patient's active cancer care treatment					
F6. Being solely responsible for the patient's primary care management upon the completion of the patient's active cancer care					
F7. Being solely responsible for the primary care management of older adult cancer survivors who have been "cancer free" for 5 years					
F8. Being responsible for cancer disease-specific, tumor surveillance and the monitoring for cancer treatment-related adverse effects/events of older adult cancer survivors who have been "cancer-free" for 5 years					

E16. How likely would your fellowship program be willing to fund/send its geriatric medicine fellows who are attending an AGS annual scientific meeting to an in-depth, 4½-hour geriatric oncology-focused preconference workshop — taking place in the afternoon of the day preceding the meeting?

□ Highly likely□ Likely□ Not Sure□ Unlikely□ Highly unlikely

F. Clinical roles for geriatricians in the care of older cancer patients.

What is your level of agreement <i>with regard to appropriate clinical roles of geriatricians and other geriatrics practitioners within the cancer care paradigm?

F9. In addition to the above, are there other appropriate clinical roles for geriatricians and other geriatrics practitioners *within the cancer care paradigm?*

Yes → No

If "Yes": Please list.

F10. In your opinion geriatricians and geriatrics practitioners are best suited in which of the following role(s) in relation to their clinical roles within the cancer care paradigm?

□ Consultative model only
□ Primary care model only
□ Both consultative and primary care models
□ There is no role for geriatricians and geriatrics practitioners.

You have completed the survey.
Did you find any of the questions unclear or difficult to answer?
Yes
No
If "Yes": Please list the numbers of unclear or difficult questions.
Comments (Optional):
Thank you for your time and effort.

Geriatric education utilizing a palliative care framework

Beverly Lunsford and Laurie Posey

ABSTRACT

The dramatic growth of persons older than age 65 and the increased incidence of multiple, chronic illness has resulted in the need for more comprehensive health care. Geriatrics and palliative care are medical specialties pertinent to individuals who are elderly, yet neither completely addresses the needs of older adults with chronic illness. Interprofessional faculty developed Geriatric Education Utilizing a Palliative Care Framework (GEPaC) to teach an integrated approach to care. Interactive online modules use a variety of instructional methods, including case-based interactive questions, audiovisual presentations, reflective questions, and scenario-based tests. Modules are designed for online education and/or traditional classroom and have been approved for Continuing Medical Education. Pre- and posttest scores showed significant improvements in knowledge, attitudes, and skills. Participants were highly satisfied with the coursework's relevance and usefulness for their practice and believed that GEPaC prepared them to address the needs of older adults for disease and symptom management, communicating goals of care, and supportive/compassionate care.

Introduction

The average life expectancy of Americans has increased steadily from 68 in 1950 to 78 years in 2007 (Arias, 2011). As people live longer, they are more likely to experience chronic health conditions. In fact, more than 75% of people older than age 65 have multiple chronic conditions, and the average 75-year-old lives with three chronic health conditions (Anderson, 2010). As the number of chronic conditions increase, the percentage of people who experience activity limitations also increases proportionately, from 4% experiencing limitations with no chronic conditions, 15% with one, 28% with two, 43% with three, 52% with four, and 67% with five (Anderson, 2010).

Although some people may die quickly and predictably, the time spent living with chronic conditions is often prolonged with intermittent illness, progressive loss of functioning over several years, and diminished quality of life. To live as fully and as long as possible, older adults with multiple chronic illnesses need high-quality health care with supportive and coordinated care beginning early in diagnosis (Lynn, 2001). In addition, older adults want to communicate their values and treatment preferences with their

Color versions of one or more of the figures in the article can be found online at www.tandfonline.com/wgge.

families and health care providers, and they need the opportunity to anticipate and prepare for potential disability and even death, while continuing to treat their disease. To address the complex needs of older adults, an innovative educational intervention was developed that integrated the best tenets of geriatric care and palliative care. This article describes the development, implementation and evaluation of an online interactive education program, Geriatric Education Utilizing a Palliative Care Framework (GEPaC) that prepares interdisciplinary health care professionals to meet the special needs of older adults with serious, chronic, and/or life-threatening illnesses and their families.

Background

Geriatrics model

The field of geriatrics addresses the health concerns of older people with a focus on disease and problems associated with advancing age. Geriatrics includes maintaining the health, independence, and quality of life as defined by each person using the collaborative efforts of an interdisciplinary team (e.g., occupational therapy, physical therapy, speech therapy, physicians, nurses, nurse practitioners, and physician assistants).

Palliative care model

In addition to the general geriatric approach, palliative care provides specific attention to the needs of people who are not necessarily dying in the predictable future from their disease, but who are experiencing significant disease burden from progressive illness. Palliative care seeks to relieve suffering, control symptoms, and restore or maintain functional capacity. Palliative care also recognizes that aging, and eventually dying, are natural processes and focuses on providing a comfortable and meaningful period of time according to the individual's own values and preferences (National Consensus Project, 2008). Like geriatrics, palliative care utilizes an interdisciplinary team approach, and palliative care emphasizes the individual and family as members of the team.

Toward an integrated geriatrics and palliative care model

An integrated geriatrics and palliative care model was needed to address functional needs, symptom management, and suffering in physical, psychological, social and spiritual dimensions, especially as comorbid diseases become more burdensome to the individual and family. GEPaC offers a greater focus on the family as the unit of care, highlighting communication and shared decision making around the individual's unique goals of care. This model is consistent with the work of Morrison and Meier (2003), experts in geriatrics and palliative care, who edited the first *Geriatric Palliative Care* in 2003 to educate health care professionals in an integrated approach to geriatrics and palliative care.

The GEPaC curriculum consists of evidence-based modules developed by an interdisciplinary team of health educators under the direction of the authors. The modules provide information on concepts, assessments, and interventions to be used with this vulnerable population and describe the cultural shift from a traditional curative or disease management model of chronic illness care to a more integrated model. The curative and disease-modifying approach to care focuses on life sustaining treatment. As medical treatments fail and the individual becomes more debilitated and dependent, referrals may be made for palliative measures. Eventually individuals will be provided with a terminal diagnosis and may be referred for hospice care until their death. There is a definite shift from providing curative/disease-modifying care to only providing hospice and end-of-life care. However, there are problems with this model of care as many chronic, life-limiting conditions do not follow a linear path of decline. Moreover, palliative measures that promote quality of life are often a valuable adjunct to disease-modifying care. Further, what might be viewed as curative treatments may also provide palliative benefits and should not be discontinued if the goal of care is comfort and supportive care.

The alternative and integrated model of care that is taught in the GEPaC modules allows for the flexibility of curative and disease-modifying care to coexist with palliative measures. Over time, as disease-modifying measures provide less benefit, there is a natural shift to increased emphasis on palliation. Ideally, individuals will enter hospice when the primary goals of care are focused on palliation and they have been given a terminal diagnosis (which by Medicare guidelines is fewer than 6 months to live). Unlike the traditional shift from curative and disease-modifying care to hospice care, palliative care may be offered from the time of diagnosis of serious, chronic illness along with disease-modifying care, gradually increasing as the ability to treat the disease decreases. This integrated model is particularly important for older adults with multiple chronic illnesses, which are not curable, but are associated with symptoms, such as pain, dyspnea, gastrointestinal maladies, and functional capacity, that can be addressed to improve quality of life.

Development of the GEPaC curriculum

The interdisciplinary GEPaC curriculum was developed in an online, modular format to provide a flexible and adaptable means of educating interdisciplinary students and professionals practicing in different health care settings. It was designed to be used in traditional classroom and nontraditional learning settings (i.e., online, self-paced, and continuing education). With an emphasis on critical thinking and problem solving, case studies were developed to reflect various complex, real-world practice situations and engage collaborative, interdisciplinary thinking from the various health care practice areas. GEPaC employs multiple instructional strategies to engage learners, including audiovisual presentations, interactive diagrams and flowcharts, case-based learning, reflective questions, and scenario-based pre- and posttests.

An eight-person interdisciplinary faculty team representing medicine, nursing, advanced practice nursing, physician assistants, and counseling followed a systematic instructional design process to conceptualize and develop the interactive modules. This model, known as ADDIE (analysis, design, development, implementation, and evaluation), is a standard approach for developing instructional materials, including interactive, online learning modules (Schlegel, 1995). See Figure 1.

During the analysis phase, the goals of the project were reviewed and discussed. The contributions of each team member were essential to ensure that the various professional roles of each discipline, including the unique, but often overlapping roles of different disciplines, were accurately and inclusively represented in the curriculum. The faculty came to consensus on the critical elements of an integrated model for geriatric and

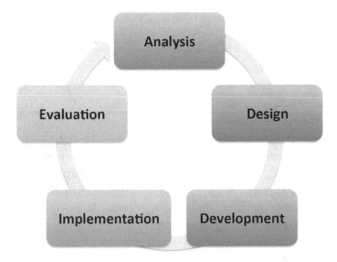

Figure 1. The analysis, design, development, implementation, evaluation (ADDIE) model: A systematic instructional design approach.

palliative care: (1) Introduction to GEPaC, (2) Person- and Family-Centered Care, (3) Communication, (4) Interdisciplinary Collaboration, (5) Multidimensional Aspects of suffering, and (6) Quality of Life. These elements were evidence- and theoretically based. The resulting model provided a framework for developing goals and learning objectives for each instructional module during the high-level design phase. Based on this work, the team decided upon the overarching curriculum structure with modular design approach that included an overview module to introduce learners to the framework and separate "deeper dive" modules to teach each critical element in detail. Once developed, the GEPaC online course was made available to students and practitioners globally through an open-access learning management system (LMS). Learners self-registered through the LMS, and the system tracked their progress, enabling self-paced completion over time.

GEPaC Modules

The GEPaC curriculum consists of six online modules that include actual stories of older adults; and the modules use case studies, videos, and/or audio recordings to illustrate the concepts. Module 1, Geriatric Palliative Care: An Integrated Approach, provides an overview of the need for an integrated geriatric and palliative care approach due to the epidemiology of chronic illness in the older adult and the impact on functional status and quality of life. The module discusses the framework for the education program and describes the integration of the clinical, functional goals-oriented focus of geriatrics with the supportive, quality of life focus of palliative care.

Module 2, Person- and Family-Centered Care, discusses the evidence-base for a person and family-centered approach to care that facilitates more informed health care decision making for older adults and families facing serious, chronic illness. A case study of an older adult with dementia illustrates a person-centered approach to care. The roles of various interdisciplinary health care professionals are discussed in relation to a person- and family-centered approach to care of older adults and their families with recognition of critical transition points during health and illness that facilitate the decision-making process and anticipatory guidance.

Module 3, Communication, discusses the importance of viewing communication as a process in the care of older adults and their families for effective health care decision making that includes health status review, treatment options, decision -making and goal setting, advance care planning, preferences, and changes in condition. This module also examines the critical communication issues of discussing bad news, dealing with family conflicts, and evaluating diminished cognitive capacity for health care decision making. Three different health care scenarios are presented with audio of actors playing the roles of health care professionals, an older adult, and several family members. The scenarios illustrate the application of the setting up, perception, invitation, knowledge, emotions, and strategies (SPIKES) communication model for breaking bad news (Baile et al., 2000) and a 10-step model for effective communication and goal setting within patient and family meetings (Weissman, Quill, & Arnold, 2010). Best practices are offered for the ongoing process of goal setting, advance care planning, and addressing family conflicts with older adults and their families or partners, along with advance care planning tools and documents that clinicians may offer individuals and families during this planning process.

Module 4, Interdisciplinary Collaboration, discusses the challenges of interdisciplinary collaboration and offers strategies to facilitate the integration of team functioning. This module presents the evidence-based benefits of interdisciplinary collaboration for improving safety and patient outcomes for older adults. A video of a team meeting that includes a physician, nurse, physician assistant, occupational therapist and social work counselor illustrates at least five key concepts for effective interdisciplinary collaboration: valuing inquiry and dialog; recognizing personal and organizational biases; discussing assumptions, goals, and values; and summarizing disparate ideas.

Module 5, Multidimensional Approach to Suffering, uses a case study to discuss the multifaceted aspects of pain and suffering for older adults and their families. The case evolves as an older woman experiences the loss of her husband, considers the possibility of living with her daughter's family, experiences a severe fall, and eventually finds community housing to meet her particular needs. The module emphasizes the aspects of suffering and the importance of using a person-centered approach for determining the effect on the individual and his or her meaning of the experience. The module includes evidence-based assessments, interventions, and evaluations to effectively manage the physical, psychological, social, and spiritual aspects of suffering that are contextualized to an older adult's needs and quality of life. Opportunities are provided for interactive decision making about the use of pharmacologic, nondrug, and complementary interventions for pain and symptom management.

The final module, Quality of Life, focuses on supporting older adults and their families with critical issues that affect their health, ability to cope, and death and bereavement. The quality of life framework developed by Ferrell, Hassey Dow, and Grant (1995) provides a multidimensional model to assess and understand each person as a unique bio-psycho-social spiritual being who is complex in nature, and who varies in his or her processes of growth and development. The stories of four different individuals and their families illustrate how empowered decision making, fostering hope and enabling a sense of control contribute to quality of life. In addition, they show how the diverse values, preferences, and beliefs people have may influence how they view what is important for quality of life.

Usability testing of the modules was conducted with 13 graduate nursing student volunteers who were enrolled in a teaching with technology course. They provided feedback on the content, design, and workability of the interactive modules that resulted in improvements for timing of slides and interactive features, and select content revision. After revisions were completed, the GEPaC modules were disseminated as widely as possible for health care professionals and others working to improve care for older adults and their families. Dissemination vehicles included professional conferences, a geriatric education website and newsletters, and national organizations in hospice and palliative care. The completed GEPaC modules were approved for 6.5 hours of Continuing Medical Education credit by the National Hospice and Palliative Care Organization (NHPCO) and made accessible on the NHPCO website for use by health care professionals. Modules 1 through 5 were made available for open access on January 15, 2013, and Module 6 was released in June 2013.

Education evaluation design and method

Sample

Learners logged into the LMS using a self-created user-name and password. With Institutional Review Board approval, learners completed the pretests prior to completing each module, and posttests and evaluation surveys upon completion. Learners' test scores and responses were recorded by the LMS and later exported for statistical analysis. A single score was assigned for each pretest and posttest, and scores could range from 1 to 100 points. Module 1 had five questions worth 20 points each. All the other modules had 10 questions worth 10 points each. From January 15, 2013 to February 16, 2015, modules were completed by 416 learners from multiple professional disciplines, including nursing ($n = 243$), social work ($n = 42$), medicine ($n = 19$), occupational therapy ($n = 5$), public health ($n = 3$), physical therapy ($n = 5$), other ($n = 20$), and not reporting ($n = 79$).

There were a total of 243 different learners and 58% of the learners held a baccalaureate or master's degree. The learners with a doctoral degree were nursing ($n = 16$), medicine ($n = 7$), and other ($n = 2$). Learners with a masters' degree included nursing ($n = 50$), social worker ($n = 15$), physical therapy ($n = 2$), medicine ($n = 2$), occupational therapy ($n = 2$), public health ($n = 1$) and other ($n = 5$). Learners reporting a baccalaureate degree were nursing ($n = 55$), social worker ($n = 1$), physical therapy ($n = 2$), public health ($n = 2$) and other ($n = 4$). Learners with associates degree and/or diploma were nurse ($n = 30$) and other ($n = 1$). There were several learners ($n = 47$) who did not report education level or profession.

The Palliative Care Network, an international platform to teach, interact, and exchange ideas for palliative care professionals, disseminated the modules. Learners included clinicians from the United States, as well as eight from six countries, including the Netherlands, Argentina, Canada, India, Lithuania, and South Africa.

Evaluation

Pre- and posttests were utilized to evaluate the effectiveness of the modules in teaching the integrated geriatric and palliative care approach. Faculty developed the test questions based on the objectives for each module. Module 1 had five questions and the other modules contained 10 questions. The pre- and posttest questions were the same for each module. The pre- and posttest questions are available by logging in to the online modules or by contacting the author. No feedback was provided to the learners based on their pretest responses, however, remedial or reinforcing feedback was provided based on posttest responses. Learners also completed an evaluation of each module to indicate the relevance and usefulness of the knowledge and skills in clinical practice using a Likert-type scale of *strongly agree* (5) to *strongly disagree* (1).

Results

The actual number of people taking the modules varied: M1 (N = 214), M2 (N = 133), M3 (N = 118), M4 (N = 89), M5 (N = 105), and M6 (N = 51). Learners were free to complete any of the modules in any sequence and were awarded continuing education credit upon successful completion of each individual module. About one-half of the learners who completed the first module also completed M2, M3, and M5. Differences in knowledge from pre- to posttest were statistically significant (p > .05) (Table 1).

Results of learner perception of relevance and usefulness of the knowledge and skills in clinical practice indicated that the modules increased their overall knowledge of the subjects; were relevant to their job functions; could be immediately applied in practice; would improve their job performance/competence; were sound, credible, and nonbiased; and used effective teaching strategies (Table 2).

Discussion

The GEPaC curriculum addressed a critical need in health care to improve the care of older adults with serious chronic illness. The curriculum was based on a new model for integrating geriatrics and palliative care and can be used by faculty in courses that teach these concepts. The online format allows for flexible delivery of modules, such as independent continuing education independent study followed by classroom discussion, or traditional classroom presentation.

GEPaC teaches a new model for improving care of older adults experiencing chronic illness using an interdisciplinary approach that addresses the special needs associated with aging, as well as palliative care for chronic illnesses that can cause increasing functional loss, frailty, and cognitive impairment. This approach is consistent with Morrison (2013) who described palliative care as interdisciplinary care that focuses on relieving suffering and achieving optimal quality of life, for individuals and their caregiver. When the

Table 1. Analysis of geriatric education utilizing a palliative care framework pre- and posttest scores

Module	Difference in mean	t	df	Significance (2-tailed)
M1: Geriatric Palliative Care: An Integrated Approach	−8.22	−7.01	213	.000*
M2: Person- and Family-Centered Care	−13.91	−8.71	132	.000*
M3: Communication	−4.83	−6.07	117	.000
M4: Interdisciplinary Collaboration	−34.27	−15.91	88	.000
M5: Multidimensional Aspects of Suffering	−22.48	−13.26	104	.000
M6: Quality of Life	−26.21	−9.37	50	.000

*p < .05.

Table 2. Mean ratings for evaluation factors[a]

	Module 1		Module 2		Module 3		Module 4		Module 5		Module 6	
	n	M	n	M	n	M	n	M	n	M	n	M
The course increased my overall knowledge in the subject.	202	4.2	125	4.3	110	4.4	80	4.1	98	4.4	44	4.3
The course was relevant to my area of practice job function.	202	4.6	125	4.5	109	4.5	81	4.3	98	4.5	44	4.4
I will be able to directly and immediately (i.e., within 1 month) apply what I learned in this course to my professional practice job function.	200	4.3	124	4.3	109	4.4	80	4.1	98	4.3	44	4.2
The information I learned in this course will improve my competence and performance in my professional practice job function.	201	4.2	125	4.3	110	4.4	80	4.1	98	4.4	43	4.4
The course was sound, credible and nonbiased.	200	4.0	124	4.0	110	4.0	78	4.0	95	4.0	44	4.0
The teaching strategies utilized for this course were effective.	200	4.3	125	4.4	110	4.4	80	4.1	98	4.4	44	4.3

a. The percent total does not equal 100%, as 18% of participants did not report their educational level.

individual is an older adult, the nature and duration of disease may differ from the younger population, as older adults frequently develop and live with one or more chronic diseases for many years. Lynn & Adamson (2003) advocated that the end of life must be viewed as a period of life that spans several years, not just weeks or months. Thus, palliative care must be thoroughly integrated with conventional geriatric medical care, rather than viewed as separate specialties.

Since the first textbook on geriatric palliative care (Morrison & Meier, 2003), Morrison has advocated for building the evidence-base for palliative care in older adults. The GEPaC is an evidence-based curriculum for palliative care of older adults, especially in relation to pain and symptom management, and enhancing quality of life. The integration of evidence-based, practice-relevant instruction with real-world examples, case-based learning, and critical thinking challenges resulted in an engaging and effective set of online materials for educating interdisciplinary practitioners worldwide. The quality and effectiveness of the modules has been supported by significant improvement in participants' pre- and posttest scores, and highly positive feedback from learner evaluations.

Limitations

The nonexperimental pre/post test design limits the generalizability of the results. There was no comparison group, and it is possible that improvements on posttest scores are due to previous exposure to the questions on the pretest. In addition, though participants reported satisfaction with the learning experience and indicated the learning would be applicable to practice, these findings were self-reported. There was no objective measure of transfer to the practice environment.

Conclusion

As the U.S. and global populations shift to a greater percentage of older adults, 76% who have chronic illness, there is a concomitant increase in the need for clinicians who can address the unique needs of older adults with serious illness. Clinicians need the knowledge, skills and attitudes to address the needs of older adults experiencing the uncertainty and complexity of living with multiple chronic, and sometimes life-threatening, illnesses. The integration of geriatrics and palliative care models of care can help engage older adults and their family in health care decision making and address issues that affect their quality of life.

This evaluation of the GEPaC modules was quantitative and limited in scope. Further rigorous evaluation, including qualitative data to examine how learners are actually using the information to improve care for older adults with chronic illness and their families, is needed. It would also be important to explore how faculty are using the curriculum in classrooms, clinical, and/or other continuing education arenas. Additional research could determine how the modules could be improved and expanded to address additional concerns of learners.

Acknowledgments

The authors want to acknowledge the following faculty and scholars who contributed to the development of the GEPaC modules:

- Cheryl Arenella MD, MPH, Health Care Consultant, The Corridor Group
- Jacqueline Barnett, MSHS, PA-C, Assistant Professor, Department of Physician Assistant Studies, School of Medicine and Health Sciences, GW
- Philip Blatt, PT, PhD, NCS; Adjunct Instructor, Department of Physical Therapy and Health Care Sciences, School of Medicine and Health Sciences, GW
- Elizabeth Cobbs, MD; Chief of Geriatrics & Extended Care, Washington DC VAMC & Professor of Medicine, GW
- Mary Corcoran, PhD, OTR/L, FAOTA, Associate Dean for Faculty Development for Health Sciences, School of Medicine and Health Sciences, GW
- Laurie Lyons, MA, Director of Instructional Technology and Design of Health Sciences Programs, School of Medicine and Health Sciences, GW
- Paul Tschudi, Ed.S, MA, LPC, Lecturer, Graduate School of Education and Human Development; Military Advisor and Counselor, School of Nursing, GW

Funding

This project was supported by the Health Resources and Services Administration (HRSA) of the U.S. Department of Health and Human Services (HHS) under grant number 5-D62-10-001 Geriatric Education Utilizing a Palliative Care Framework, $500,000. This information or content and conclusions are those of the author and should not be construed as the official position or policy of, nor should any endorsements be inferred by HRSA, HHS or the U.S. Government.

References

Anderson, G. (2010, February). *Chronic care: Making the case for ongoing care* Princeton, NJ: Robert Wood Johnson Foundation. Retrieved from www.rwjf.org/pr/product.jsp?id=50968
Arias, E. (2011, September 28). Life expectancy by age, race, and sex: Death-registration states, 1900–1902 to 1919–1921, and United States, 1929–1931 to 2007 [Table 11] *United States life tables, 2007. National Vital Statistics report.* Hyattsville, MD: U.S. Department of Health and

Human Services, National Center for Health Statistics, Center for Disease Control. Retrieved from http://www.cdc.gov/nchs/data/nvsr/nvsr59/nvsr59_09.pdf

Baile, W. F., Buckman, R.., Lenzi, R., Glober, G., Beale, E. A., & Kudelka, A. P. (2000). SPIKES – A six step protocol for delivering bad news: Application to the patient with cancer. *Oncologist, 5*, 302–311. doi:10.1634/theoncologist.5-4-302

Ferrell, B. R., Hassey Dow, K., Grant, M. (1995). Measurement of the quality of life in cancer survivors. *Quality of Life Research, 4*, 523–31.

Lynn, J. (2001). Perspectives on care at the close of life. Serving patients who may die soon and their families: The role of hospice and other services. *Journal American Medical Association, 285*, 925–932. doi:10.1001/jama.285.7.925

Lynn, J., & Adamson, D. (2003, June 14). *Living well at the end of life, adapting health care to serious chronic illness in old age* (Rand Health White Paper WP-137). RAND Health. Retrieved from http://www.medicaring.org/whitepaper/

Morrison, R., & Meier, D. (Eds). (2003). *Geriatric palliative care.* New York, NY: Oxford University Press.

Morrison, R. S. (2013). Research priorities in geriatric palliative care: An introduction to a new series. *Journal of Palliative Medicine, 16*(7), 726–729. doi:10.1089/jpm.2013.9499

National Consensus Project. (2008). *Clinical practice guidelines for quality palliative care.* Brooklyn, NY: National Consensus Project for Quality Palliative Care. Retrieved from http://www.aacn.org/WD/Practice/Docs/CP_Guidelines_for_Quality_Palliative_Care.pdf

Schlegel, M. J. (1995). *A handbook of instructional and training program design.* ERIC Document Reproduction Service ED383281. Retrieved from http://files.eric.ed.gov/fulltext/ED383281.pdf

Weissman, D., Quill, T., & Arnold, R. (2010, February). The family meeting: Starting the conversation #223. *Journal of Palliative Medicine, 13*(2), 204–205. doi:10.1089/jpm.2010.9878

Improving health care student attitudes toward older adults through educational interventions: A systematic review

Linda Ross, Paul Jennings, and Brett Williams

ABSTRACT
Educational institutions should aim to positively influence the attitudes of future health care practitioners toward older patients to ensure the provision of quality patient care. This systematic review of the literature aims to determine the effectiveness of educational interventions designed to improve health care student behaviors and/or attitudes toward older people. The 29 studies included in this review utilized a variety of interventions, methods, and measurement tools. The most common type of educational intervention incorporated interaction with real patients. Few studies evaluated the impact of interventions on behavior; therefore, more observational studies are required. Overall interventions incorporating interactions with real patients who are independently living had a positive impact on student attitudes toward older adults. Clinically focused placements with patients who are ill may still have a place in the development of the patient-centered interview and assessment skills, along with improving confidence and competence, despite not having a favorable impact on attitudes.

Introduction

Quality and compassionate care should be the aim of all health care practitioners. To achieve this they must have not only an understanding of patient conditions and needs, but also have the attitude and willingness to provide such care. This is important with all patients, particularly older patients. Not only are older adult populations increasing around the globe, this group is more susceptible to declining health and independence (Oeppen & Vaupel, 2002). Excluding practitioners specializing in younger population groups, it is evident that current health care students will encounter large numbers of older patients, and that these patients will have varied and often multiple biopsychosocial conditions (Denton & Spencer, 2010; Vaupel, 2010). As attitudes are associated with quality of patient care (Chambers & Ryder, 2009; Cornwell & Goodrich, 2009; Courtney, Tong, & Walsh, 2000; Haidet et al., 2002; Hanson, 2014; Holroyd, Dahlke, Fehr, Jung, & Hunter, 2009) it is important to investigate how we are preparing our future practitioners to care for patients in this important and unique group.

Attitudes have long been associated with behavior. Ajzen's (1991) theory of planned behavior (TPB) suggests a causal relationship between attitudes, intentions, and behavior.

According to this theory, attitudes toward an object or group, such as older adults, will influence intentions and ultimately behaviour toward them. Positive attitudes toward older adults translates to favorable behavior toward them, whereas the opposite is true for negative attitudes. A meta-analysis of 185 independent empirical tests investigating the efficacy of the TPB provided support for the theory as a predictor of intentions and behaviour (Armitage & Conner, 2001). Although measuring behavior directly would provide the best evidence of behavior, this is challenging due the difficulties associated with measuring behavior. As an alternative, attitudes, which ultimately influence behavior, and have been shown as a predictor of intention, are a much more practical alternative for researchers to measure.

As attitudes influence intentions and behavior this then translates to patient care and outcomes. Negative or stereotypical attitudes toward older patients are associated with behaviors that negatively affect their care (Chambers & Ryder, 2009; Cornwell & Goodrich, 2009; Courtney et al., 2000; Haidet et al., 2002; Hanson, 2014; Holroyd et al., 2009). Stereotypical attitudes can reduce the likelihood of individualized care with all older adults regarded as being the same and therefore treated the same (Victor, 2010). Holding such views can also impair the health care providers' ability to accurately and impartially assess patients and their needs (Taylor, 2005). Views regarding older adults as weak, forgetful, or lacking independence can lead to behavior that perpetuates such traits and can also lead to undignified care (Baillie, 2007; Courtney et al., 2000). Examples of such behavior include speaking in a patronizing manner, using loud and childish speech, and making derogatory comments (Bond, Peace, Dittmann-Kohli, & Westerhof, 2007). Unfortunately poor patient care often borders on and can progress to neglect, mistreatment, and abuse. A recent systematic review of elder mistreatment in nursing homes found widespread issues ranging from psychological mistreatment such as failure to provide adequate social stimulation, violations of rights, inappropriate restraint, all the way through to physical neglect and abuse (Lindbloom, Brandt, Hough, & Meadows, 2007). Although elder abuse is a much broader issue and can result from a combination of numerous factors including role modeling, workloads, and staffing shortages, attitudes toward older patients can also play a role.

Educational institutions should aim to positively influence the attitudes of future health care practitioners toward older patients to ensure the provision of quality patient care. Attitudes toward older adults can be best affected by increasing knowledge, awareness, and understanding (Hanson, 2014; Mellor, Chew, & Greenhill, 2007). Although foundation concepts can be taught using traditional didactic means, attitudes require an alternate approach. Kolb's (2014) experiential learning theory (ELT) is often used as a basis for how students learn and develop attitudes. The ELT asserts that learning occurs from the learner being in touch with the realities of what they are studying. It involves direct sense experience and in-context action like fieldwork, service learning, or problem-based learning, where learners are able to contextualize and reflect on what they have previously learnt (Kolb, 2014). A more personalized learning journey allows students to develop their own beliefs, values, and attitudes based on their own experiences and reflections.

Driven by the need to deliver quality health care to an increasing population of older adults, numerous studies have evaluated health care professional attitudes and the impact of education and experience on these. This systematic review of the literature aims to determine the effectiveness of educational interventions designed to improve health care student behaviors and/or attitudes toward older people.

Method

A systematic review was conducted in March 2016 in accordance with the Preferred Reporting Items for Systematic Reviews and Meta-Analyses (PRISMA) Statement (Moher, Liberati, Tetzlaff, & Altman, 2009). An electronic search of EMBASE, CINAHL, MEDLINE, PsychINFO, ERIC, Google Scholar, and ProQuest was conducted. The search strategy was developed by the authors in conjunction with a library database specialist. Medical subject headings, key words, phrases, and synonyms describing health care students, educational interventions, and attitudes/behavior toward older people were combined and searched. A full list of search terms is available in Figure 1. Following duplicate removal studies were screened and excluded based on title and abstract. The full texts of remaining studies were reviewed against the inclusion/exclusion criteria independently by two authors. Disagreements were discussed and final inclusion was decided by mutual agreement. A search of references and citations of identified papers was also conducted to source any additional studies from the identified articles.

	Healthcare student		Educational intervention		Behaviour &/or attitudes
1	Students, Health Occupations (MeSH)	26	Education (MeSH)	45	Attitude of Health Personnel (MeSH)
2	Emergency medical technicians (MeSH)	27	Education, Medical, Undergraduate (MeSH)	46	Health Knowledge, Attitudes, Practice (MeSH)
3	Nutritionists (MeSH)	28	Education, Nursing, Baccalaureate (MeSH)	47	Behavior*
4	Nurses (MeSH)	29	Teaching (MeSH)	48	Attitud*
5	Physicians (MeSH)	30	Educat*	49	Aged (MeSH) (49-54 limited to Title & Abstract)
6	Social Workers (MeSH)	31	Teach*	50	Age*
7	Physical Therapists (MeSH)	32	Instruct*	51	Elder*
8	healthcare	33	Pedago*	52	Older adult*
9	health adj1 care	34	Method*	53	Older patient*
10	paramedic*	35	Approach*	54	Older people
11	emergency medical technician	36	Technique*	55	45 or 46 - 48
12	nurs*	37	Strateg*	56	49 or 50 - 54
13	Physician*	38	Innovat*	57	55 & 56
14	Doctor*	39	Intervention*		
15	social adj1 work*	40	Program*	58	25 & 44 & 57
16	speech adj1 therap*	41	Design*	59	Limit 2000 – current & English
17	physiotherap*	42	26 or 27 - 33		
18	physical adj1 therap*	43	34 or 35 - 41		
19	occupational adj1 therap*	44	42 & 43	*Truncation	
20	Student*				
21	Undergrad*				
22	20 or 21				
23	2 o r3 - 19				
24	22 and 23				
25	1 or 24				

Figure 1. MEDLINE search strategy. MeSH = Medical Subject Heading.

Inclusion criteria

Studies that described the effectiveness of educational interventions designed to improve health care student attitudes and/or behavior toward older adults were included. Undergraduate health care students from medicine, nursing, social work, paramedicine, speech therapy, physiotherapy, occupational therapy, or nutrition and dietetics were included. Although this is not an all-encompassing list of health care students, agreement was reached among the authors that the selected professions shared common traits and would encounter large numbers of older patients in their practice. Educational interventions or combinations of strategies that were single sessions or over multiple sessions and time frames were eligible. They may have included, but were not limited to, didactic methods, simulation, clinical placements, case studies, service learning, workshops, and /or gamification. Peer-reviewed quantitative, qualitative, or mixed-methods studies utilizing either validated tools or alternative approaches to evaluate student attitudes and/or behavior were also eligible. Only studies available in English and published after the year 2000 were included. It was considered studies beyond this date would include the most contemporary educational interventions.

Exclusion criteria

Studies involving health care students from disciplines beyond those detailed above, or from postgraduate courses were not eligible. It was considered postgraduate students would introduce too much heterogeneity due to potential experience in the workforce. Studies evaluating an entire curriculum/course were ineligible as it would be difficult to ascertain discrete components or interventions that were responsible for results. Also ineligible were studies not evaluating and reporting student attitudes/behavior toward older adults at all, or where this was not the predominant aim of the study.

Data extraction

Data including authors, year, location, study design, population, intervention, attitude/ behavior measures and psychometric properties, and results was extracted from eligible articles and tabulated. Two authors discussed and reached agreement on the final content. Statistical significance of results was indicated where available, with effect size and power calculations reported or calculated from available statistics where possible.

Quality assessment and impact

The Medical Education Research Study Quality Instrument (MERSQI) was utilized to assess the selected studies for quality. MERSQI is designed to measure the methodological quality of education research studies and has been tested for reliability and validity (Reed et al., 2007). Studies were scored for quality out of 18 with the exception of two solely qualitative studies that were scored out of 15 (points relating to measure validity were not applicable). Kirkpatrick's levels were (Yardley & Dornan, 2012) applied to assess the educational impact of interventions used in the selected studies. This tool comprises four levels of evidence that are tangible, easily measured outcomes of education (1 = participation, 2a = attitudes, 2b = knowledge/skills, 3 = behavior, 4a = organizational benefit,

4b = benefit to patients) (Yardley & Dornan, 2012). Studies were assessed independently by the authors. Differences in interpretation were discussed until consensus was reached.

Data synthesis and analysis

A narrative synthesis was used due to the heterogeneity of study methods and measures. Results were synthesised according to study methodology and intervention type. Randomised control, nonrandomized control, and quasiexperimental studies were grouped and results between intervention and control groups were analyzed. Pre- and poststudy designs were also grouped and results pre- and postintervention were analyzed. Studies were also grouped by intervention type for further analysis. A thematic approach was utilized to synthesize and analyze the qualitative results. Two authors reviewed the qualitative data independently and reach agreement on the final themes for inclusion.

Results

Included studies

An initial search of seven databases resulted in 3,781 studies. Following the removal of duplicates, 3,362 studies remained. A review of title and abstracts left 177 studies. A full-text review of these against the inclusion/exclusion criteria left 25 studies for inclusion. Four more articles were identified through a search of citations and references. The final number of studies included for data extraction and analysis was 29. A study selection overview is shown in Figure 2 (Moher et al., 2009).

Data extraction

The 29 included studies are summarized in Table 1. The majority of studies were conducted in the United States (19), followed by Canada (3), China (2), and one each from Australia, Ireland, Netherlands, Switzerland, and New Zealand. Most studies employed quantitative (16) or mixed methods (11); only two were solely qualitative. Health care professions studied included medicine (18), nursing (9), social work (4), physiotherapy and nutrition (3 each), and occupational therapy and paramedics (one each). Study designs varied as follows: randomized controlled pre–post (3), randomized controlled post only (1), controlled pre–post (12), pre–post (11) and post only (2).

A number of quantitative measurement tools were used to assess attitudes, these included the Aging Semantic Differential (ASD; Rosencranz & McNevin, 1969) (11), Kogan's Attitudes Towards Old People Scale (KAOP; Kogan, 1961) [4], University California at Los Angeles Geriatric Attitudes Scale (UCLA-GAS; Reuben et al., 1998) [4], Maxwell-Sullivan's Attitudes Scale (MSAS; Maxwell & Sullivan, 1980) [3], and various other newly developed and yet-to-be-validated surveys were used on single occasions. Behavior was measured on only two occasions with the use of a patient-centered interview objective structure clinical examination (OSCE; Harden & Gleeson, 1979), and the Students' Caring Behaviour Scale (SCBS; Hwang et al., 2013). Attitudes were also assessed via the following qualitative means: written reflections (6), focus groups (4) and free text questions (2).

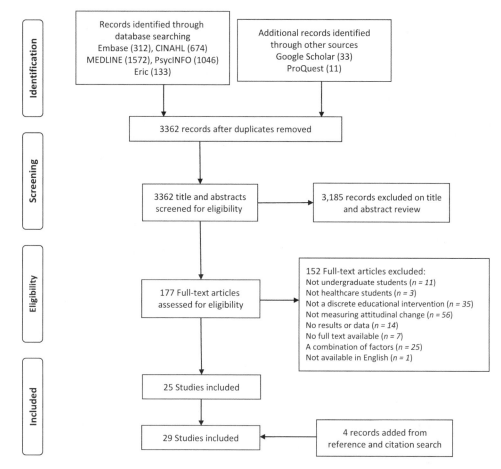

Figure 2. Search results.

Interventions were grouped into four distinct themes. The most common intervention utilized was interaction with real patients (18). These included interventions such as senior mentor programs, service learning, home visits, community interaction activities, and interviews. The second most common intervention type was using sensory activities, such as the Aging Game and Geriatrix (6). A variety of workshop or module activities were used in three studies. Two interventions had a clinical focus.

Quality assessment and impact

MERSQI scores ranged from 8 to 14.5/18 with an average score of 10.5/18. The qualitative studies each scored 7/15. The majority of the quantitative/mixed studies scored 10 or greater (78%). The randomized controlled studies averaged a MERSQI of 12/18, the nonrandomized controlled 11/18, and the pre–post 10/18. The six studies utilizing sensory activities averaged a MERSQI of 10.5/18, the two clinical focus interventions 13/18, whereas the three workshop interventions and the 18 interaction with real patient's interventions averaged 10/18.

Table 1. Included studies.

	Study (Author & year)	Location	Study design	Population (n) & participation requirements	Intervention	Attitude measure & psychometric properties (If report for study cohort)	Method	Kirkpatrick	MERSQI
1	Basran et al. (2012)	Canada	Pre-post (T3–1 year)	PT, Med, Nurs, Nut, Pharm, SW (141) Voluntary -elective	Senior Mentor Program Teams of 3/4 IPE students partnered with IL (4 visits)	ASD (Polizzi), FG	Mixed	2a	10.5
2	Beauvais et al. (2015)	United States	Controlled, Pre-post	Nurs (134) Mandatory	Service Learning IG—2 × 6-hr guided sessions (n = 66) CG—2 × 6-hr clinical placements (n-68)	KAOP	Quant	2b	11.5
3	Bernard et al. (2003)	United States	Controlled, pre-post	Med (225) Mandatory	Senior Mentor Program IG—Partnered with IL (4 x visits) (n = 117) CG—not reported (n = 108)	ASD	Quant	2a	11
4	Cohen et al. (2004)	United States	Post only	SW (45) Mandatory	Focus Groups (60–90 minute) With IL (n = 15) With service providers (n = 30)	Written reflection	Qual	2a	7[a]
5	Corwin et al. (2006)	United States	Post only	Med (36) Mandatory	Senior Mentor Program Partnered with IL (4–6 × visits)	FG	Qual	2a	7[a]
6	Denton et al. (2009)	United States	Controlled, pre-post	Med (33) Voluntary	Home visits IG—home visits, online materials, discussion (n = 16) CG—online materials only (n = 17)	Attitudinal survey, Written reflection	Mixed	2b	10.5
7	Diachun et al. (2006)	Canada	RCT, post x 2 (T2–1 year)	Med (42) Mandatory	Sensory Activity IG—3-hr sensory experiential activity (n = 25) CG—3-hr didactic (n = 17)	FAQ (Bias score), Free text	Mixed	2b	10.5
8	Diachun et al. (2010)	Canada	RCT, pre-post	Med (191) Mandatory	Geriatric Placement IG—elder care rotation (n = 108) CG—standard placement (n = 74)	UCLA-GAS, PCI OSCE	Quant	3	14.5
9	Dorfman et al. (2002)	United States	Controlled, pre-post	SW (47) Mandatory	Service Learning IG—Partnered with AL (4 × visits) (n = 13) CG—not reported (n = 34)	Attitudinal scales, (α = .54—.67 & .60 —.72), Free text Q's, Written reflections	Mixed	2a	7.5
10	Duke et al. (2009)	United States	Pre-post	Med (55) Mandatory	Senior Mentor Program 2-hr lecture SMP (4 x 45 min visits with AL)	UCLA-GAS, Written reflection	Mixed	2a	10
11	Eskildsen & Flacker (2009)	United States	Pre-post	Med (129) Mandatory	5 Day module—interactive, small group format + interview with an older adult advancing in age each day	UCLA-GAS, FAQ (Bias score)	Quant	2a	10.5
12	Fitzgerald et al. (2006)	United States	Controlled, pre-post	Med, Nurs, Pharm, SW (50) Mandatory	4-day program IG—Interdisciplinary geriatric care (n = 32) CG—(n = 18)	UCLA-GAS, (α = .61), MSAS, (α = .54)	Quant	2a	10.5
13	Furze et al. (2008)	United States	Pre-post	Nurs, OT, PT, Pharm (64), Voluntary	Community-based learning IP teams of 4 partnered with AL	SAAS, FG, Written reflective	Mixed	2a	8
14	Goeldlin et al. (2014)	Switzerland	Controlled, pre or post	Med (147) Mandatory	Geriatric clinical skills training—4 × 2.5 hr (real patients) IG—posttest (n = 76) CG—pretest (n = 71)	UCLA-GAS	Quant	2b	11.5

(Continued)

Table 1. (Continued).

Study (Author & year)	Location	Study design	Population (n) & participation requirements	Intervention	Attitude measure & psychometric properties (If report for study cohort)	Method	Kirkpatrick	MERSQI
15 Henry et al. (2007)	United States	Pre-post	Nut, PT, CA (N = 156) Voluntary	Aging game (shortened)	ASD (Polizzi), (α = .94 & .96)	Quant	2a	10.5
16 Henry et al. (2011)	United States	RCT, pre-post	Nurs, Nut (124) Mandatory	Aging game IG—90 min aging game (n = 51) CG—75 min tutorial (n = 47)	ASD (Polizzi), (α = .91), Written reflections	Mixed	2a	12
17 Hwang et al. (2013)	China	Pre-post, longitudinal (T3—16 months)	Nurs (126) Mandatory	Service learning 6 hrs preservice training 6 x visits with AL or nursing homes or veteran homes	SCBS, (α = .93), R-KAOP, (α = .81)	Quant	2b	11.5
18 Lee et al. (2008)	United States	Controlled, pre or post	Nut (100) Mandatory	Interviews IG—3 x visits with IL (n = 52) CG—3 x visits with young adult (n = 48)	WOAI, (α = .75 & .82), Written reflection	Mixed	2a	12
19 Leung et al. (2012)	China	RCT, pre-post (T3—1 month)	Med, Nurs (103) Voluntary	Service learning IG—Half-day workshop Met OA 1-2 hrs/week x 10 weeks Intergenerational sharing session (n = 48) CG—aging online SDL (n = 55)	KAOP	Quant	2a	12
20 Lu et al. (2010)	United States	Controlled, Pre-post	Med (137) Voluntary	Senior Teacher Education Partnership IG—Home visits with IL (n = 46) CG—(n = 91)	ASD, (α = .92), FG	Mixed	2a	11
21 Robinson & Rosher (2001)	United States	Pre-post	Med (49) Not stated	Half-full Aging Simulation Experience—presentation and simulation experience	ASD	Quant	2a	8.5
22 Ross & Williams (2015)	Australia	Pre-post	Para (11) Voluntary	Community-Interaction Activity with IL	ASD, FG	Mixed	2a	9.5
23 Ryan et al. (2007)	Ireland	Pre-post T2-1 year	Nurs (94) Mandatory	Home visits with IL (10 in year) Theory sessions	KAOP, (α = .80 & .81)	Quant	2a	10.5
24 Shue et al. (2005)	United States	Controlled, pre-post	Med (161) Mandatory	Senior Mentor Program	ASD, (α = .95 & .93), MSAS, (α = .84 & .87)	Quant	2a	11
25 van de Pol et al. (2014)	Netherlands	Controlled, pre-post	Med (53) Voluntary	Geriatrix game IG—4 weeks in combination with didactic (n = 29) CG—4-week, not geriatric specific—didactic only (n = 24)	ASD	Quant	2b	11
26 Varkey et al. (2006)	United States	Pre-post	Med (84) Mandatory	Aging game	ASD, MSAS	Quant	2a	10.5
27 Walsh et al. (2008)	United States	Controlled, pre-post	Nurs (28) Voluntary	Home visits IG—Creative-Bonding Intervention (n = 11) CG—Friendly Visit (n = 11)	R-KAOP, (α = .80 & .85)	Mixed	2a	10

#	Author	Country	Study design	Profession (n)	Mandatory/Voluntary	Intervention	Measure	Type	Quality	Score
28	Westmoreland et al. (2009)	United States	Pre-post (Half students pre/half past)	Med (247)	Mandatory	Workshop— Prereflection, introduction, council of elders (75 min dialogue with IL, postreflection)	GAS	Mixed	2a	9.5
29	Wilkinson et al. (2002)	New Zealand	Controlled Pre-post	Med (186)	Mandatory	Home visits IG—Interview in pairs IL (n = 41) & AL (n = 40) CG—visits young adults (n = 105)	ASD (Polizzi)	Quant	2a	10

Note. FG = focus group; AL = assisted living older adults; IL = independent living older adults; IG = intervention group; CG = control group; IP = interprofessional; PCI = patient centered interview; OSCE = objective structured clinical examination; ASD = Aging Semantic Differential (Modified—Polizzi, 2003); KAOP = Kogan's Attitudes Towards Older People Scale; FAQ Bias Score = Facts on Aging Quiz; UCLA-GAS = University of California at Los Angeles Geriatric Attitudes Scale; MSAS = Maxwell-Sullivan's Attitude Scale SCBS = Students' Caring Behavior Scale; WOAI = Wall-Oyer Aging Inventory ; GAS = Geriatrics Attitudes Scale; SAAS = Survey of Attitudes on Aging Scale; PT = physical therapy; Med = medicine; Nut = nutrition & dietetics; Pharm = pharmacy; SW = social work; IPE = interprofessional education; Para = paramedic; RCT = Randomized Control Trial; SMP = Senior Mentor Program; OT = occupational therapy; CA = care administration; SDL = self-directed learning.

α = Cronbach alpha (≥ .70 acceptable), Wash out stated in study design if not immediately after intervention.

a. Qualitative studies scored out of 15 only.

Kirkpatrick's levels of education outcomes ranged for 2a to 3. The majority (n = 22, 76%) were level 2a (attitudes). One study (3%) achieve a level 3 (behavior) whereas the remaining (n = 6, 21%) were level 2b (knowledge and/or skills). Although knowledge acquisition was not included in the aims of this review, several studies incorporated measures of this domain in addition to attitudes and/or behavior, and this was therefore accounted for in the quality assessments.

Quantitative data synthesis

An analysis of the results of 13 studies comparing intervention and control groups are presented in Table 2. Four studies employing these methods were excluded from this table due to insufficient data to compare groups postintervention.

Of the four randomized studies, only one reported improved attitudes in the intervention group in comparison to the control group, however the effect was small and not statistically significant (Henry, Ozier, & Johnson, 2011). Two studies showed declining attitudes in the intervention groups (Diachun, Dumbrell, Byrne, & Esbaugh, 2006; Diachun, van Bussel, Hansen, Charise, & Rieder, 2010), whereas another found improved attitudes in the control group were greater than that of the intervention group (Leung et al., 2012).

Of the nine controlled/quasiexperimental studies three reported statistically significant improvement in the intervention group in comparison to the control group (Bernard, McAuley, Belzer, & Neal, 2003; Denton et al., 2009; Lee & Waites, 2006). In Bernard et al. (2003) insufficient data was provided to determine the effect size and power, Denton et al. (2009) had a large effect size (0.78) but was underpowered at 0.54, Lee, Hoerr, Weatherspoon, and Schiffman (2008) had a medium effect size (0.30) and was also underpowered at 0.32.

An analysis of the results of 14 studies comparing pre- and postintervention results are presented in Table 3. Eleven of the studies showed some improvement in attitudes postintervention. Only five however had statistically significant results, with three having a large effect size. Basran et al. (2012) reported the most favorable results between Time 1 and Time 2, but these were not sustained at Time 3 (12 months). Several studies included subscale analysis for the ASD rather than totals. These studies reported statistically significant improvements in attitudes in at least two out of three subscales (Ross & Williams, 2015; Varkey, Chutka, & Lesnick, 2006; Wilkinson, Gower, & Sainsbury, 2002).

Two studies, though designed to improve and measure attitudes, had predominantly clinically focused interventions. Goeldlin et al. (2014) achieved a MERSQI of 11.5 and found attitudes improved postintervention (p = .06). Diachun et al. (2010) achieved a MERQI of 14.5 (the highest score of all studies) and found the control and intervention groups attitudes worsened; slightly less in the intervention group (p = .09). Diachun et al. was also one of only two studies to measure behavior. The intervention group had statistically significant higher results (p < .001), and a pass rate of 95% versus 78% (p < .001) on a patient-centered interview OSCE with a geriatric focus (Diachun et al., 2010).

Three studies used workshop type interventions. Eskildsen and Flacker (2009) had a MERSQI of 10.5 and found improvement in attitudes postintervention (p < .001). Westmoreland et al. (2009) had a MESQI of 9.5 and also found improvement in attitudes

Table 2. Attitude results (between groups—intervention vs control).

Author	Tool	Intervention or control	Type of intervention	N	Pre M (SD)	Post	Post 2	Attitude direction	d	p	Power
Randomized control studies											
Diachun et al. (2010)	UCLA-GAS	Intervention	Geriatric placement	108	3.72 (0.42)	3.58 (0.44)		↓	0.24	0.09	46%
		Control	Standard placement	74	3.69 (0.43)	3.46 (0.55)		↓			
Henry et al. (2011)	ASD (Polizzi)	Intervention	Aging Game	51	74.08 (19.58)	68.59 (15.16)		↑	0.07	0.21	23%
		Control	Tutorial	47	75.68 (17.70)	69.62 (15.59)		↑			
Leung et al. (2012)	KOAP	Intervention	Service learning	48	45.04 (6.48)	57.26 (5.21)	45.83 (20.88) (1 month)	↑	0.12	0.44	52%
		Control	Online SDL	55	43.72 (5.84)	57.28 (6.34)	47.18 (8.97) (1 month)	↑			
Randomised (post only)											
Diachun et al. (2006)	FAQ (Bias)	Intervention	Sensory activity	25	Not measured	−3.50 (2.54)	−4.58 (1.74) (12mths)	↓	0.46	0.65	87%
		Control	Didactic	17	Not measured	−4.06 (2.16)	−3.94 (2.22) (12 months)	↑			
Controlled/quasi-experimental studies											
Beauvais et al. (2015)	KOAP	Intervention	Service learning	66	130.76 (10.5)	137.33 (11.1)		↑	0.05	NA	NA
		Control	Clinical placement	68	136.47 (10.6)	136.69 (13.4)		↑			
Bernard et al. (2003)	ASD	Intervention	Senior mentoring program	117	3.45	3.05		↑	NA	0.002	NA
		Control	Not reported	108	3.42	3.25		↑			
Denton et al. (2009)	Attitudinal survey	Intervention	Home visits	16	81.8 (0.16)	Reported 9.8% increase		↑	0.78	0.04	54%
		Control	Online material	17	84.6 (0.16)	Reported 0.5% increase		↑			
Dorfman et al. (2002)	Attitudinal scales	Intervention	Service learning	13	2.88 (0.29)	3.32 (0.29)		↑	0.62	0.07	52%
		Control	Not reported	34	2.91 (0.36)	3.11 (0.38)		↑			
Fitzgerald et al. (2006)	UCLA-GAS	Intervention	Interdisciplinary program (4 day)	32	4.0 (0.4)	4.1 (0.4)		↑	0.0	0.72	72%
		Control	Not reported	18	Not reported	4.1 (0.4)		↓			
Goeldlin et al. (2014)	UCLA-GAS	Intervention	Geriatric clinical skills training	76	Not reported	51		NA	NA	0.06	NA
		Control	Not reported	71	49			↑			
Lee et al. (2008)	WOAI	Intervention	Interviews with IL	52	3.45 (0.35)	3.58 (0.42)		↑	0.30	< 0.05	32%
		Control	Visits with young adults	48	3.49 (0.39)	3.45 (0.44)		↓			
Lu et al. (2010)	ASD	Intervention	Home visits	46	116.17 (18.01)	107.93 (23.26)		↑	0.34	0.12	62%
		Control	Not reported	91	118.70 (19.26)	115.07 (18.18)		↑			
Shue et al. (2005)	MSAS	Intervention	Senior mentoring program	72	62.02 (8.19) MSAS	66.50 (5.67) MSAS		↑	0.43	0.19	92%
		Control	Standard program	89	Not measured	64.03 (5.71)		NA			

Note. UCLA-GAS = University California at Los Angeles Geriatric Attitudes Scale; ASD = Aging Semantic Differential; KOAP = Kogan's Attitudes Towards Older People Scale; SDL = Self-directed Learning; FAQ = Facts on Aging Quiz; WOAI = WallOyer Aging Inventory; MSAS = Maxwell-Sullivan's Attitude Scale. Statistically Significant: $p < .05$; Effect size: d = Cohen's d—0.2 (small), 0.3 (medium), 0.5 (large); Power ≥ 80%.

Studies providing insufficient antintervention results to compare groups were excluded from this table.

Table 3. Attitude results (within groups).

Author	Tool	Type of intervention	N	Pre M (SD)	Post	Post 2	Attitudinal direction	d	p	Power
Basran et al. (2012)	ASD (Polizzi) 80 year old man	Senior mentoring program	111	78.71 (16.76)	66.54 (19.27)	~73 (from bar graph) (12 months)	↑	0.67	<0.001	100%
	ASD (Polizzi) 80 year old woman		113	69.47 (15.47)	56.61 (18.87)	~63 (from bar graph) (12 months)	↑	0.74	< 0.001	100%
Duke et al. (2009)	UCLA-GAS	Senior mentoring program	55	16.11 (3.98)	14.24 (5.17)		↑	0.40	0.004	49%
Eskildsen & Flacker (2009)	UCLA-GAS	5-day module	129	3.7	3.8		↑	NA	< 0.001	NA
Furze et al. (2008)	SAAS	Community based learning	64	Not reported	Not reported		↑	NA	NA	NA
Henry et al. (2007)	ASD (Polizzi)	Aging game	156	78.84 (18.2)	82.61 (20.7)		↓	0.19	< 0.001	18%
Hwang et al. (2013)	KOAP	Service Learning AL	43	107.25 (1.73)	109.60 (1.71)	113.58 (1.69) (16 months)	↑	3.7	<0.01	100%
		Service Learning NH	40	102.67 (1.63)	104.8 (1.35)	100.95 (1.70) (16 months)	↓	1.0	<0.05	100%
		Service Learning VH	43	101.39 (1.81)	103.90 (1.68)	98.97 (1.40) (16 months)	↓	1.6	<0.001	100%
Robinson & Rosher (2001)	ASD	Aging simulation experience	49	123.35	116.14		↑	NA	NA	NA
Ross & Williams (2015)	ASD	Community interaction activity	11	NA	NA	NA	↑	NA	NA	NA
Ryan et al. (2007)	KAOP	Home visits	94	126.4 (9.99)	128.0 (9.54)		↑	0.16	0.33	87%
van de Pol et al. (2014)	ASD	Geriatrix game	29	84 (11)	77 (15)		↑	0.52	0.02	74%
Varkey et al. (2006)	ASD	Aging game	84	NA	NA	NA	↑	NA	NA	NA
Walsh et al. (2008)	KAOP	Friendly visits	11	80.73	67.37		↑	NA	0.03	NA
Westmoreland et al. (2009)	GAS	Workshop	247	NA	NA	NA	↑	NA	NA	NA
Wilkinson et al. (2002)	ASD (Polizzi)	Interviews with IL & AL	41	NA	NA	NA	↑	NA	NA	NA

however did not provide a statistical analysis. Fitzgerald et al. (2006) found no difference between the control and intervention group ($p = .72$).

Six studies used sensory activities as their intervention. Henry, Douglass, and Kostiwa (2007) and Diachun et al. (2006), both with a MERSQI of 10.5, showed a decline in attitudes postintervention ($p < .001$, $p = .65$, respectively); (Diachun et al., 2006; Henry, Douglass, & Kostiwa, 2007) The other four studies showed improved attitudes with only Henry et al. (2011) and van de Pol et al. (2014) providing data ($p = .21$, $p = .02$, respectively) (Henry et al., 2011; Robinson & Rosher, 2001; van de Pol et al., 2014; Varkey et al., 2006).

Eighteen studies used interactions with real patient as the intervention. Of the 16 employing quantitative methods all reported improved attitudes, eight of which were statistically significant with MERSQI scores ranging from 10 to 12. Three of these, Basran et al. (2012), Denton et al. (2009), and Hwang, Wang, and Lin (2013) also had large effect sizes ($p < .001$, $d = .67$; $p = .04$, $d = 0.78$; $p < .01$, $d = 3.7$, respectively). Duke, Cohen, and Novack (2009) and Lee et al. (2008) had medium effect sizes ($p = .004$, $d = .40$; $p = .05$, $d = .30$, respectively). Beauvais, Foito, Pearlin, and Yost (2015), Bernard et al. (2003), and Walsh, Chen, Hacker, and Broschard (2008) did not report or provide adequate data to calculate effect size ($p = .05$, $p = .002$, and $p = .03$, respectively).

Behaviour was measured and reported in only two studies. Hwang et al. (2013) used a self-report Students Caring Behaviour Scale and found statistically significant increases in caring scores at postintervention and follow-up. Diachun et al. (2010) observed behavior via a patient-centered interview with an older patient. They found the intervention group scored significantly higher and had significantly higher pass rates than the controlgroup.

Qualitative data synthesis

The studies incorporating qualitative analysis overwhelmingly reported positive findings. The most commonly reported themes were, students were able to learn about older adults' lives, their capabilities, challenges, and needs. Students also gained an increased awareness of and reduced their own beliefs about myths and stereotypes associated with older people. Other themes including negative attitudes are displayed in Table 4.

Discussion

Twenty-nine studies were identified and analyzed to determine the effectiveness of educational interventions designed to improve health care student behaviors and/or attitudes toward older people. These studies incorporated a variety of study designs and interventions.

Interaction with real patients

The 18 studies incorporating interactions with real patients included service learning, senior mentor programs, and home visits. These interventions were essentially experiential in nature but also had numerous other factors in common that differentiate them from traditional clinical placements. Each involved interaction with older patients who were independently living and high functioning. This is in contrast to the ill, frail and dependent nursing home or hospital patients students can come into contact with during traditional clinical placements. Although a balanced interaction with a variety of patients is preferable to provide realistic expectations of older adults, encounters with predominantly patients who are ill and older has been shown to instil negative stereotypes and beliefs (Fitzgerald, Wray, Halter, Williams, & Supiano, 2003). In addition, in each of these studies, the aim of the interaction was to develop an understanding and awareness of older patients and to practice interpersonal communication skills.

Table 4. Qualitative results summary.

Attitudinal themes	Basran et al. (2012)	Cohen et al. (2004)	Corwin et al. (2006)	Denton et al. (2009)	Diachun et al. (2006)	Dorfman et al. (2002)	Duke et al. (2009)	Furze et al. (2008)	Henry et al. (2011)	Lee et al. (2008)	Lu et al. (2010)	Ross & Williams (2015)	Walsh et al. (2008)	Westmoreland et al. (2009)	
Learned about older adults lives—capabilities, challenges, needs	x	x	x	x	x		x	x	x	x	x	x			11
Increased awareness and reduced myths & stereotypes	x	x	x	x	x	x	x	x	x	x	x	x		x	12
Wise and experienced; can learn from them		x				x		x		x	x			x	6
Individuals—physical, mental, attitude			x			x	x	x	x	x				x	7
Ability to see things from patients perspective									x						1
Like to talk and often lack this interaction													x		1
Demanding on others														x	1
Set in their ways												x			1
Poor hearing, poor memory, frustrating							x	x							2

All 18 studies cited improved attitudes postintervention in comparison to control groups. Basran et al. (2012), one of the most promising studies, saw 111 students from various disciplines showing improved attitudes postparticipating in a senior mentoring program ($p < .001$, $d = .67$). Students in this program met with a senior mentor on four occasions and followed discussion guidelines for each visit as follows: "general history"; "living situation and changing world"; "medication, nutrition, and physical activity"; and "unstructured social event." Students were also required to complete a structure reflection during the program to complete the cycle and increase knowledge, develop skills, clarify values, analyze and apply what they have learnt as per Kolb's learning cycle (Kolb, 2014).

Other studies within this group with positive results were Hwang et al. (2013) who found nursing students interacting with well or assisted living older adults improved their attitudes ($p < .001$), however groups interacting with nursing/veteran home patients declined. This reinforces what previous research has taught us about the impact the type interaction (with ill vs. well older adults) has on attitudes (Fitzgerald et al., 2003). Duke et al. (2009) and Lee et al. (2008) found improved attitudes from a senior mentoring program and interviews with older patients and achieved a statistically significant medium effects ($p = .004$, $d = .40$; $p < .05$, $d = .30$, respectively). Denton et al. (2009) and Dorfman et al. (2002) also had positive results, however both studies used instruments not yet psychometrically appraised. Walsh et al. (2008) and Beauvais et al. (2015) had statistically significant results, however insufficient data to calculate effect size and power. Overall interventions incorporating interactions with independently living real patients had a positive impact on student attitudes towards older adults.

Sensory activities

Six studies used sensory-type activities to help students gain an understanding of what it feels like to be an older person. Three studies utilized the Aging Game, where participants experience a variety of different sensory deficits, for example, hearing and vision loss. Overall the results were not conclusive either way. Henry et al. (2007) conducted a pre–post study using a shortened version of the Aging Game in 2007 and found results worsened ($p < .001$, $d = .19$). In 2011 Henry then conducted a randomized control study using the full Aging Game and found attitudes improved in the intervention and control groups (who participated in a tutorial) ($p = .21$, $d = .07$) (Henry et al., 2011b). The third study (Varkey et al., 2006) utilizing the Aging Game cited improved attitudes postintervention but provided no statistical analyses or findings.

Two of the other studies using other sensory activities had major flaws in study design. Diachun et al. (2006) found the control groups' attitudes improved but the intervention group worsened. This was based on two posttests, one directly after the intervention and one at 12 months. No pretest was conducted and the measure of attitudes was the Facts on Aging Quiz bias score that has been discredited as a measure of attitudes (Holtzman & Beck, 1979). Robinson and Rosher (2001) cited improved attitudes but did not provide enough data to evaluate. A third study (van de Pol et al., 2014) utilized the Geriatrix Game and found improved attitudes ($p = .02$, $d = .52$), this was however a very small study with only 29 participants.

Despite the fact that four out of the six studies utilizing sensory activities had some improvement in attitudes the study design, quality, lack of reported data makes it impossible to form a conclusion about the effect of this type of intervention. As these sensory interventions that could actually perpetuate the myths and stereotypes associated with older people questions need to be raised about their ultimate impact on attitudes. They may in fact improve understanding, knowledge, and empathy while reinforcing negative stereotypes. The full impact these types of interventions have on behavior is not actually known as this was not measure in these studies.

Workshops

Three studies used workshops or modules as the intervention to improve attitudes and/or behaviour. Eskildsen and Flacker (2009) and Westmoreland et al. (2009), pre–post studies, showed improved attitudes. Eskildsen and Flacker incorporated an interview with a progressively aging simulated patient over the 5-day largely didactic program. They reported improvement in attitudes postintervention ($p < .001$), however the change appeared to be very small (effect size and power was unable to be calculated due to insufficient data) (Eskildsen & Flacker, 2009). Westmoreland et al. (2009) incorporated a discussion with elders into a 90-minute workshop on aging. Although they cited improved attitudes they presented item analysis only and no overall data was presented to support this (Westmoreland et al., 2009).

The Fitzgerald et al. (2006) study intervention incorporated four interdisciplinary workshops focusing on geriatric assessment and care. This study had small numbers and found no difference between the control and intervention groups.

Although there is some support for this type of intervention the reported studies do not warrant a favorable conclusion that this type of intervention improves attitudes or behavior. Of interest, however, is that though presenting traditional workshop/module learning interventions they all also incorporated the use of real or simulated patients into their programs.

Clinical focus

The two studies in this category use interventions involving interacting with real patients, however the focus was on clinical assessment and treatment. Diachun et al. (2010) used geriatric clinical clerkships for medicine students as the intervention and measured knowledge and skills, as well as attitudes. Goeldlin et al. (2014) used geriatric skills training with medical students and measured attitudes only. Although Goeldlin et al. found attitudes improved postintervention ($p = .06$), there were numerous flaws in the study design and reporting of results. The investigators used different cohorts for the pre- and postmeasures and reported insufficient data to calculate power and effect size.

Diachun et al. (2010), a well-designed randomized control study (MERSQI = 14.5) found the control and intervention groups attitudes worsened, slightly less in the intervention group ($p = .09$). Importantly, the intervention was conducted in geriatric medical and psychiatric units exposing participants to predominantly older people who were "ill." Diachun et al. was, however, one of only two studies to measure behavior via a patient-centered interview OSCE with a geriatric focus. The intervention group had higher results, and pass rate ($p < .001$) . Even though the attitudes results were not statistically significant, in combination with the behavior results they raise some interesting discussion points. It appears that this intervention (geriatric clinical placements) decreased attitudes while improving behavior. This goes against Ajzen's (1991) TPB supposing that improved attitudes leads to improved behavior. Perhaps the answer lies in the effect exposure to patients who are older, lower functioning, and ill has on attitudes. Most research suggests this has a negative influence on the attitudes of health care students (Allan & Johnson, 2008; Bousfield & Hutchison, 2010; Fitzgerald et al., 2003; Schwartz et al., 2001). This intervention did however give students experience and confidence in conducting a patient-centered interview and assessment of older adults which was reflected in the development of improved skills and behavior.

Limitations

The lack of objective measures of attitudes and behavior was a limitation. Most studies evaluated attitudes using self-report measures. These measures are subject to social desirability bias and not as reliable subjective observational measures (van de Mortel, 2008). Only one study used a subjective observational measure to evaluate behavior. Finally the analysis and synthesis of heterogeneous studies is extremely challenging. This required a narrative approach to result in synthesis and subjective decisions about the grouping of studies for analysis.

Recommendations for future research

The findings of this review, in combination with previous research, highlight the importance of the type of older patients students are interacting with and the impact this has on attitudes. More studies similar to Hwang et al. (2013) that evaluated the attitudes of student placements with older patients of differing health and independence levels are necessary to better understand the ramifications of this. More research is also needed to evaluate to effectiveness of sensory activities such as the Aging Game. There were insufficient quality studies in this review to form any conclusions about the effectiveness. Finally more observational studies are required to evaluate the effect interventions have on behaviour and patient care.

Conclusion

Educational interventions designed to improve health care student attitudes and/or behavior toward older adults varied in their effectiveness. The evaluated studies varied greatly in study design, quality, and intervention type. The most common and successful intervention type was those utilizing interaction with real patients. When these interactions were with real patients who were living independently the impact on student attitudes was positive. Clinically focused placements with patients who are ill may still have a place in the development of patient-centered interview and assessment skills, along with improving confidence and competence, despite not having a favorable impact on attitudes. Sensory activities also have value in raising awareness and empathy for patients who are older, yet further investigation is required to better understand the impact on attitudes and behavior.

References

Ajzen, I. (1991). The theory of planned behavior. *Organizational Behavior and Human Decision Processes, 50*(2), 179–211. doi:10.1016/0749-5978(91)90020-T

Allan, L. J., & Johnson, J. A. (2008). Undergraduate attitudes toward the elderly: The role of knowledge, contact and aging anxiety. *Educational Gerontology, 35*(1), 1–14. doi:10.1080/03601270802299780

Armitage, C. J., & Conner, M. (2001). Efficacy of the theory of planned behaviour: A meta-analytic review. *British Journal of Social Psychology, 40*(4), 471–499. doi:10.1348/014466601164939

Baillie, L. (2007). The impact of staff behaviour on patient dignity in acute hospitals. *Nursing Times, 103*(34), 30–31.

Basran, J. F., Dal Bello-Haas, V., Walker, D., MacLeod, P., Allen, B., D'Eon, M., ... Trinder, K. (2012). The longitudinal elderly person shadowing program: Outcomes from an interprofessional senior partner mentoring program. *Gerontology & Geriatrics Education, 33*(3), 302–323. doi:10.1080/02701960.2012.679369

Beauvais, A., Foito, K., Pearlin, N., & Yost, E. (2015). Service learning with a geriatric population: Changing attitudes and improving knowledge. *Nurse Educator, 40*(6), 318–321. doi:10.1097/NNE.0000000000000181

Bernard, M. A., McAuley, W. J., Belzer, J. A., & Neal, K. S. (2003). An evaluation of a low-intensity intervention to introduce medical students to healthy older people. *Journal of the American Geriatrics Society, 51*(3), 419–423. doi:10.1046/j.1532-5415.2003.51119.x

Bond, J., Peace, S. M., Dittmann-Kohli, F., & Westerhof, G. (2007). *Ageing in Society.* London, England: Sage.

Bousfield, C., & Hutchison, P. (2010). Contact, anxiety, and young people's attitudes and behavioral intentions towards the elderly. *Educational Gerontology, 36*(6), 451–466. doi:10.1080/03601270903324362

Chambers, C., & Ryder, E. (2009). *Compassion and caring in nursing.* Oxon, England: Radcliffe Publishing.

Cohen, H. L., Sandel, M. H., Thomas, C. L., & Barton, T. R. (2004). Using focus groups as an educational methodology: Deconstructing stereotypes and social work practice misconceptions concerning aging and older adults. *Educational Gerontology, 30*(4), 329–346. doi:10.1080/03601270490278858

Cornwell, J., & Goodrich, J. (2009). Exploring how to ensure compassionate care in hospital to improve patient experience. *Nursing Times, 105*(15), 14–16.

Corwin, S. J., Frahm, K., Ochs, L. A., Rheaume, C. E., Roberts, E., & Eleazer, G. (2006). Medical student and senior participants' perceptions of a mentoring program designed to enhance geriatric medical education. *Gerontology & Geriatrics Education, 26*(3), 47–65. doi:10.1300/J021v26n03_04

Courtney, M., Tong, S., & Walsh, A. (2000). Acute-care nurses' attitudes towards older patients: A literature review. *International Journal of Nursing Practice, 6*(2), 62–69. doi:10.1046/j.1440-172x.2000.00192.x

Denton, F. T., & Spencer, B. G. (2010). Chronic health conditions: Changing prevalence in an aging population and some implications for the delivery of health care services. *Canadian Journal on Aging, 29*(1), 11–21. doi:10.1017/S0714980809990390

Denton, G. D., Rodriguez, R., Hemmer, P. A., Harder, J., Short, P., & Hanson, J. L. (2009). A prospective controlled trial of the influence of a geriatrics home visit program on medical student knowledge, skills, and attitudes towards care of the elderly. *Journal of General Internal Medicine, 24*(5), 599–605. doi:10.1007/s11606-009-0945-5

Diachun, L., van Bussel, L., Hansen, K. T., Charise, A., & Rieder, M. J. (2010). "But I see old people everywhere": Dispelling the myth that eldercare is learned in nongeriatric clerkships. *Academic Medicine, 85*(7), 1221–1228. doi:10.1097/ACM.0b013e3181e0054f

Diachun, L. L., Dumbrell, A. C., Byrne, K., & Esbaugh, J. (2006). But does it stick? Evaluating the durability of improved knowledge following an undergraduate experiential geriatrics learning session. *Journal of the American Geriatrics Society, 54*(4), 696–701. doi:10.1111/j.1532-5415.2006.00656.x

Dorfman, L. T., Murty, S., Ingram, K. G., & Evans, R. J. (2002). Incorporating intergenerational service-learning into an introductory gerontology course. *Journal of Gerontological Social Work, 39*(1/2), 219–240.

Duke, P., Cohen, D., & Novack, D. (2009). Using a geriatric mentoring narrative program to improve medical student attitudes towards the elderly. *Educational Gerontology, 35*(10), 857–866. doi:10.1080/03601270902782412

Eskildsen, M. A., & Flacker, J. (2009). A multimodal aging and dying course for first-year medical students improves knowledge and attitudes. *Journal of the American Geriatrics Society, 57*(8), 1492–1497. doi:10.1111/j.1532-5415.2009.02363.x

Fitzgerald, J. T., Williams, B. C., Halter, J. B., Remington, T. L., Foulk, M. A., Persky, N. W., & Shay, B. R. (2006). Effects of a geriatrics interdisciplinary experience on learners' knowledge and attitudes. *Gerontology & Geriatrics Education, 26*(3), 17–28. doi:10.1300/J021v26n03_02

Fitzgerald, J. T., Wray, L. A., Halter, J. B., Williams, B. C., & Supiano, M. A. (2003). Relating medical students' knowledge, attitudes, and experience to an interest in geriatric medicine. *The Gerontologist, 43*(6), 849–855. doi:10.1093/geront/43.6.849

Furze, J., Lohman, H., & Mu, K. (2008). Impact of an interprofessional community-based educational experience on students' perceptions of other health professions and older adults. *Journal of Allied Health, 37*(2), 71–77.

Goeldlin, A. O., Siegenthaler, A., Moser, A., Stoeckli, Y. D., Stuck, A. E., & Schoenenberger, A. W. (2014). Effects of geriatric clinical skills training on the attitudes of medical students. *BMC Medical Education, 14*, 233. doi:10.1186/1472-6920-14-233

Haidet, P., Dains, J. E., Paterniti, D. A., Hechtel, L., Chang, T., Tseng, E., & Rogers, J. C. (2002). Medical student attitudes toward the doctor–patient relationship. *Medical Education, 36*(6), 568–574. doi:10.1046/j.1365-2923.2002.01233.x

Hanson, R. M. (2014). 'Is elderly care affected by nurse attitudes?' A systematic review. *British Journal of Nursing, 23*(4), 225–229. doi:10.12968/bjon.2014.23.4.225

Harden, R. M., & Gleeson, F. A. (1979). Assessment of clinical competence using an objective structured clinical examination (OSCE). *Medical education, 13*(1), 39–54.

Henry, B. W., Douglass, C., & Kostiwa, I. M. (2007). Effects of participation in an aging game simulation activity on the attitudes of allied health students toward older adults. *Internet Journal of Allied Health Sciences & Practice, 5*(4), 1–9.

Henry, B. W., Ozier, A. D., & Johnson, A. (2011). Empathetic responses and attitudes about older adults: How experience with the aging game measures up. *Educational Gerontology, 37*(10), 924–941. doi:10.1080/03601277.2010.495540

Holroyd, A., Dahlke, S., Fehr, C., Jung, P., & Hunter, A. (2009). Attitudes toward aging: Implications for a caring profession. *Journal of Nursing Education, 48*(7), 374–380. doi:10.3928/01484834-20090615-04

Holtzman, J. M., & Beck, J. D. (1979). Palmore's facts on aging quiz: A reappraisal. *The Gerontologist, 19*(1), 116–120. doi:10.1093/geront/19.1.116

Hwang, H.-L., Wang, -H.-H., & Lin, H.-S. (2013). Effectiveness of supervised intergenerational service learning in long-term care facilities on the attitudes, self-transcendence, and caring behaviors among nursing students: A quasiexperimental study. *Educational Gerontology, 39*(9), 655–668. doi:10.1080/03601277.2012.734159

Kogan, N. (1961). Attitudes toward old people: the development of a scale and an examination of correlates. *The Journal of Abnormal and Social Psychology, 62*(1), 44.

Kolb, D. A. (2014). *Experiential learning: Experience as the source of learning and development.* New York, NY: Pearson Education.

Lee, E.-K. O., & Waites, C. E. (2006). Infusing aging content across the curriculum: Innovations in baccalaureate social work education. *Journal of Social Work Education, 42*(1), 49–66. doi:10.5175/JSWE.2006.042110002

Lee, S.-Y., Hoerr, S. L., Weatherspoon, L., & Schiffman, R. F. (2008). Nutrition students improve attitudes after a guided experiential assignment with older adults. *Journal of Nutrition Education and Behavior*, *40*(5), 279–287. doi:10.1016/j.jneb.2007.09.011

Leung, A. Y., Chan, S. S., Kwan, C. W., Cheung, M. K., Leung, S. S., & Fong, D. Y. (2012). Service learning in medical and nursing training: A randomized controlled trial. *Advances in Health Sciences Education*, *17*(4), 529–545. doi:10.1007/s10459-011-9329-9

Lindbloom, E. J., Brandt, J., Hough, L. D., & Meadows, S. E. (2007). Elder mistreatment in the nursing home: A systematic review. *Journal of the American Medical Directors Association*, *8*(9), 610–616. doi:10.1016/j.jamda.2007.09.001

Lu, W.-H., Hoffman, K. G., Hosokawa, M. C., Gray, M., & Zweig, S. C. (2010). First year medical students' knowledge, attitudes, and interest in geriatric medicine. *Educational Gerontology*, *36*(8), 687–701. doi:10.1080/03601270903534630

Maxwell, A. J., & Sullivan, N. (1980). Attitudes Toward the Geriatric Patient Among Family Practice Residents. *Journal of the American Geriatrics Society*, *28*(8), 341–345.

Mellor, P., Chew, D., & Greenhill, J. (2007). Nurses' attitudes toward elderly people and knowledge of gerontic care in a multi-purpose health service (MPHS). *Australian Journal of Advanced Nursing*, *24*(4), 37.

Moher, D., Liberati, A., Tetzlaff, J., & Altman, D. G. (2009). Preferred reporting items for systematic reviews and meta-analyses: The PRISMA statement. *Annals of Internal Medicine*, *151*(4), 264–269. doi:10.7326/0003-4819-151-4-200908180-00135

Oeppen, J., & Vaupel, J. W. (2002). Broken limits to life expectancy. *Science*, *296*(5570), 1029–1031. doi:10.1126/science.1069675

Reed, D. A., Cook, D. A., Beckman, T. J., Levine, R. B., Kern, D. E., & Wright, S. M. (2007). Association between funding and quality of published medical education research. *Journal of the American Medical Association*, *298*(9), 1002–1009. doi:10.1001/jama.298.9.1002

Reuben, D. B., Lee, M., Davis, J. W., Eslami, M. S., Osterweil, D. G., Melchiore, S., & Weintraub, N. T. (1998). Development and validation of a geriatrics attitudes scale for primary care residents. *Journal of the American Geriatrics Society*, *46*(11), 1425–1430.

Robinson, S. B., & Rosher, R. B. (2001). Effect of the "half-full aging simulation experience" on medical students' attitudes. *Gerontology & Geriatrics Education*, *21*(3), 3–12. doi:10.1300/J021v21n03_02

Rosencranz, H., & McNevin, T. (1969). A factor analysis of attitudes toward the aged. *The Gerontologist*, *9*, 55–59.

Ross, L., & Williams, B. (2015). Real engagement improving paramedic attitudes towards the elderly. *Clinical Teacher*, *12*(1), 37–41. doi:10.1111/tct.12226

Ryan, A., Melby, V., & Mitchell, L. (2007). An evaluation of the effectiveness of an educational and experiential intervention on nursing students' attitudes towards older people. *International Journal of Older People Nursing*, *2*(2), 93–101. doi:10.1111/j.1748-3743.2007.00060.x

Schwartz, K., Joseph, P., & Simmons, L. (2001). Contact quality and attitudes toward the elderly. *Educational Gerontology*, *27*(2), 127–137. doi:10.1080/03601270151075525

Shue, C. K., McNeley, K., & Arnold, L. (2005). Changing medical students' attitudes about older adults and future older patients. *Academic Medicine*, *80*(10 Suppl), S6–9. doi:10.1097/00001888-200510001-00005

Taylor, H. (2005). *Assessing the nursing and care needs of older adults: A patient-centred approach.* Oxon, England: Radcliffe Publishing.

van de Mortel, T. F. (2008). Faking it: Social desirability response bias in self-report research. *Australian Journal of Advanced Nursing*, *25*(4), 40.

van de Pol, M. H., Lagro, J., Fluit, L. R., Lagro-Janssen, T. L., & Olde Rikkert, M. G. (2014). Teaching geriatrics using an innovative, individual-centered educational game: Students and educators win. A proof-of-concept study. *Journal of the American Geriatrics Society*, *62*(10), 1943–1949. doi:10.1111/jgs.13024

Varkey, P., Chutka, D. S., & Lesnick, T. G. (2006). The aging game: Improving medical students' attitudes toward caring for the elderly. *Journal of the American Medical Directors Association*, *7*(4), 224–229. doi:10.1016/j.jamda.2005.07.009

Vaupel, J. W. (2010). Biodemography of human ageing. *Nature, 464*(7288), 536–542. doi:10.1038/nature08984

Victor, C. R. (2010). *Ageing, health and care.* Bristol, England: Policy Press.

Walsh, S. M., Chen, S., Hacker, M., & Broschard, D. (2008). A creative-bonding intervention and a friendly visit approach to promote nursing students' self-transcendence and positive attitudes toward elders: A pilot study. *Nurse Education Today, 28*(3), 363–370. doi:10.1016/j.nedt.2007.06.011

Westmoreland, G. R., Counsell, S. R., Sennour, Y., Schubert, C. C., Frank, K. I., Wu, J., ... Inui, T. S. (2009). Improving medical student attitudes toward older patients through a "council of elders" and reflective writing experience. *Journal of the American Geriatrics Society, 57*(2), 315–320. doi:10.1111/j.1532-5415.2008.02102.x

Wilkinson, T. J., Gower, S., & Sainsbury, R. (2002). The earlier, the better: The effect of early community contact on the attitudes of medical students to older people. *Medical Education, 36* (6), 540–542. doi:10.1046/j.1365-2923.2002.01226.x

Yardley, S., & Dornan, T. (2012). Kirkpatrick's levels and education 'evidence'. *Medical Education, 46*(1), 97–106. doi:10.1111/j.1365-2923.2011.04076.x

Effect of short-term research training programs on medical students' attitudes toward aging

Dilip V. Jeste, Julie Avanzino, Colin A. Depp, Maja Gawronska, Xin Tu, Daniel D. Sewell and Steven F. Huege

ABSTRACT

Strategies to build a larger workforce of physicians dedicated to research on aging are needed. One method to address this shortage of physician scientists in geriatrics is short-term training in aging research for early-stage medical students. The authors examined the effects of two summer research training programs, funded by the National Institutes of Health, on medical students' attitudes toward aging, using the Carolina Opinions on Care of Older Adults (COCOA). The programs combined mentored research, didactics, and some clinical exposure. In a sample of 134 participants, COCOA scores improved significantly after completion of the research training program. There was a significant interaction of gender, such that female students had higher baseline scores than males, but this gender difference in COCOA scores was attenuated following the program. Four of the six COCOA subscales showed significant improvement from baseline: early interest in geriatrics, empathy/compassion, attitudes toward geriatrics careers, and ageism.

Introduction

Although the number of older Americans will increase from 15% in 2014 to 21% in 2030 (Federal Interagency Forum on Aging-Related Statistics, 2016), the gap between demand for and supply of physicians with geriatric expertise will widen (Committee on the Future Health Care Workforce for Older Americans Board on Health Care Services, Institute of Medicine, 2008). By 2030, there will be fewer than three geriatricians and less than one geriatric psychiatrist per 10,000 adults older than age 75 (American Geriatrics Society 2011; Committee on the Future Health Care Workforce for Older Americans Board on Health Care Services, Institute of Medicine, 2008; Warshaw & Bragg, 2008). By comparison, there is estimated to be one radiation oncologist per 100 adults older than age 65 needing radiation therapy in 2020 (Smith et al., 2010). Limited clinical experience in geriatrics in medical school coupled with concerns about relying on Medicare and inadequate reimbursement for geriatric services are important factors in disincentivizing a career in geriatrics; negative attitudes toward older adults may also contribute. Clinicians have pervasive negative views about seniors with medical conditions (Kearney, Miller, Paul, & Smith, 2000; Meisner, 2012). Residents and medical students are reported to provide potentially age-biased recommendations for procedures such as breast conservation or reconstruction after modified radical mastectomy (Madan, Aliabadi-Wahle, & Beech, 2001). First-year medical students endorse negative attitudes toward older adults and report low interest in geriatric medicine (Fitzgerald, Wray, Halter, Williams, & Supiano, 2003; Perrotta, Perkins, Schimpfhauser, & Calkins, 1981; Reuben, Fullerton, Tschann, & Croughan-Minihane, 1995), and only 3% to 4% of these students express a strong interest in geriatrics (Fitzgerald et al., 2003; Perrotta et al., 1981; Voogt, Mickus, Santiago, & Herman, 2008). Attitudes toward aging remain unchanged during the medical school training (Thorson & Powell, 1991). In one study of fourth-year medical students, interest in geriatrics was the third lowest among 14 specialties listed (Duthie, Donnelly, & Kirsling, 1987). Even when medical students report a moderately positive perception of older adults, 90% show an implicit preference for younger over older people (Ruiz et al., 2015).

Medical students with positive attitudes toward seniors and those who have cared for seniors prior to medical school have a greater interest in geriatrics, suggesting that interventions that reduce ageist attitudes and offer clinical geriatric experience to medical students may increase the number of physicians entering geriatrics (Fitzgerald et al., 2003). Educational programs targeted to change medical students' attitudes toward older adults lead to improved positive attitudes and reduced negative age stereotypes (Atkinson et al., 2013; Corwin et al., 2006; Laks et al., 2016; Varkey, Chutka, & Lesnick, 2006; Wilkinson, Gower, & Sainsbury, 2002; Wilson & Hafferty, 1980). Many of these interventions were designed with the goal of changing student attitudes toward aging, and not for offering aging-focused research training. There is a need for larger workforces of geriatric clinicians and researchers. Short-term research training programs, notwithstanding their limitations, are a pragmatic method for increasing the potential pipeline of physician scientists interested in aging (Jeste, Halpain, Trinidad, Reichstadt, & Lebowitz, 2007). Due to the limited time commitment required and because they can be offered early in the medical school training, these programs can involve sizable proportions of first-year medical students in research.

We evaluated the impact of two National Institutes of Health (NIH)-funded, national-level, short-term research training programs, Medical Student Training in Aging Research (MSTAR) and Medical Students' Sustained Training and Research Experience in Aging and Mental Health (M-STREAM) (Black et al., 2013; Dumbauld et al., 2014; Jeste et al., 2007), on medical students' attitudes toward aging. These programs have previously been reported to improve research self-efficacy among medical students (Black et al., 2013). A recent study by Barron, Bragg, Cayea, Durso, and Fedarko (2015) suggested highly promising longer-term results of the MSTAR program, as 7.8% of the medical students who participated in the Johns Hopkins MSTAR program between 1994 and 2010 went on to become geriatricians or were completing training to become geriatricians. This is a much higher percentage of geriatricians entering the workforce than the 0.5% of active physicians who are practicing geriatrics nationally (The Center for Workforce Studies at the Association of American Medical Colleges, 2012).

We hypothesized that participating students' attitudes toward older adults would become more positive after completing the MSTAR and M-STREAM programs. We also examined whether variation in student characteristics (e.g., gender) was associated with change in attitudes.

Method

Program description

The MSTAR and M-STREAM programs have been described previously (Black et al., 2013; Jeste et al., 2007). Briefly, MSTAR is a multisite program supported by the National Institute on Aging (NIA), American Federation for Aging Research (AFAR), and the John A. Hartford Foundation. It provides funding to several selected sites, for up to 18 first-year medical students from across the United States per site annually, to participate in an aging-focused summer research training program (8 to 12 consecutive weeks of full-time training, with stipends). M-STREAM was a single-site program, funded by the National Institute of Mental Health. M-STREAM was similar to MSTAR except that it focused on geriatric psychiatry or neuroscience research. Student selection criteria for both programs included past academic performance, interest in geriatrics or aging-related research, and potential for academic career advancement. Each selected student was paired with a research mentor in basic, clinical, or translational research, based on the student's interest, and conducted during the summer following the first year of medical school, a research project under the mentor's guidance. Students participated in didactic sessions covering topics of bioethics, effective publication strategies, and successful aging and received some clinical geriatrics exposure in other settings, primarily through a visit to a specialized geropsychiatric inpatient unit.

Study participants

University's Human Research Protections Program approved the study protocol, and informed consent was obtained from all participants. There were a total of 178 first-year medical students who completed the MSTAR and M-STREAM programs from 2011 to 2016, and 149 completed the preprogram Carolina Opinions on Care of Older Adults (COCOA) (83.7%). Data were available on demographic characteristics of all 178, and there were no differences between the 149 who completed the preprogram COCOA and the remaining 29 students in terms of gender, race/ethnicity, program, enrollment in a top-20 medical school, or project type. There were six cohorts of MSTAR students and four cohorts of M-STREAM students. Students were asked to complete several rating scales immediately prior to beginning the program and immediately following its completion. Of the 149 who completed the preprogram COCOA, 134 students completed both the pre- and postprogram COCOA. Students who only completed the preprogram COCOA were more likely to be female, $\chi^2(1) = 4.0$, $p = .046$, and a participant of the MSTAR program, $\chi^2(1) = 10.5$, $p = .001$, than those who completed both the pre- and postprogram COCOA.

Measurements

We used the COCOA (Hollar, Roberts, & Busby-Whitehead, 2011), a standardized and validated scale with strong interitem reliability (Cronbach's alpha = .811) for assessment of medical and health professional students' attitudes toward older adults. COCOA is a 42-item survey that contains six subscales: Early Interest in Geriatrics, Empathy/Compassion, Attitudes toward Geriatrics Careers, Ageism, Clinical and Social Services for Older Adults, and Social Value of Older Adults. Each item is scored on a 1 to 5 Likert-type agreement scale

Table 1. Sample questions from the Carolina Opinions on Care of Older Adults (COCOA).

COCOA Subscale	Sample Questions
Early Interest in Geriatrics	I have spent time caring for an older friend or family member.
Empathy/Compassion	I always take the time to listen to what older adults have to say.
	I would stop what I was doing and immediately help an older patient.
Attitudes toward Geriatrics Careers	Working in geriatrics might limit my lifestyle and career goals more than working in other healthcare specialties.
Ageism	Most older adults are relatively inactive and stay close to home.
Clinical and Social Services for Older Adults	It is important that healthcare providers directly help older patients understand and make joint decisions on their healthcare options.
Social Value of Older Adults	Older adults are valuable contributors to our society.

from 1 to 5, yielding total scores from 42 to 210. Higher scores reflect more positive attitudes toward seniors. The COCOA has been used in several studies to date (Atkinson et al., 2013; Biese et al., 2011; Laks et al., 2016). Table 1 illustrates sample questions from the COCOA.

Students' gender, race/ethnicity, and current medical school were obtained from their program applications. Student race/ethnicity was categorized as White, African American, Hispanic/Latino, Asian, Native Hawaiian/Other Pacific Islander, Multi-Racial, or Other. Given the small cell size, these categories were then grouped as either White or Not White, and students who identified as Multi-Racial and Other were not included in the latter grouping. Top-20 medical schools were defined by the 2015 U.S. News Best Medical Schools for Research rankings (Best Graduate Schools 2015, 2014). The research project each student completed was categorized by the program staff as basic, clinical, or translational research. Seven of the projects could not be categorized due to being unclear or mixed.

Statistical analysis

Descriptive statistics were run to describe characteristics of the total sample. Linear regression and t tests were used to determine baseline differences in preprogram COCOA scores by student characteristics, whereas paired t test was employed to determine pre- and postprogram differences in COCOA total and subscale scores. Linear regression was also used to assess for significant interactions between changes in COCOA scores and student characteristics such as gender, with the difference between the post- and preprogram scores as dependent variable and student characteristics, preprogram scores, and their interactions as independent variables. We employed a backward elimination procedure to remove redundant variables to improve parsimony and then examined significant variables ($p < .05$) in the final model. Multicollinearity among covariates was assessed using the variance inflation factor (VIF). To ensure valid inference, distribution-free methods such as the asymptotic and permutation tests were used for outcomes that exhibited severe departures from the normal distribution (Effron & Tibshirani, 1993; Tang, He, & Tu, 2012). The α level was set at .05. All statistical analyses were two-tailed.

Results

A majority of the participating students were female, White, from top-20 medical schools, enrolled in MSTAR, and completed clinical research projects (Table 2). Higher preprogram COCOA scores were associated with being female, White, enrollment in MSTAR,

Table 2. Baseline sample characteristics and preprogram Carolina Opinions on Care of Older Adults (COCOA) scores (N = 149).

Characteristic (Number)		COCOA Total Mean Score[a] (SD)	t- or F Score (df)	p Value
Gender	Female (83)	156.7 (16.8)	4.24 (1, 147)	.041
	Male (66)	150.9 (17.6)		
Race/ethnicity	White (55)	158.1 (17.4)	4.68 (1, 147)	.032
	Non-White (94)	151.8 (17.0)		
Program	MSTAR (80)	159.9 (14.0)	21.29 (1, 147)	<.001
	M-STREAM (69)	147.5 (18.5)		
Medical school Enrollment	Top 20 (75)	149.2 (18.1)	13.35 (1, 147)	<.001
	Under top 20 (74)	159.2 (15.1)		
Project-type[b]	Basic (29)	156.1 (18.0)	3.18 (2, 139)	.044
	Clinical (92)	151.8 (17.6)		
	Translational (21)	161.9 (12.5)		

Note. MSTAR = Medical Student Training in Aging Research; M-STREAM = Medical Students' Sustained Training and Research Experience in Aging and Mental Health.
[a]COCOA Total Score range = 42 to 210; COCOA Items 1, 5, 7, 8, 9, 11, 12, 13, 18, 24, 25, 26, 27, 29, 30, 32, 33, 34, 36, 37, 39, 40, and 42 are reverse-scored.
[b]Seven of the projects could not be categorized due to being unclear or mixed.

and completing translational (rather than clinical) research projects. Students from top-20 medical schools had lower COCOA scores than others.

Overall, there was a significant improvement in total COCOA scores from pre- to postprogram (Table 3). Four of the six COCOA subscales showed significant improvement from pre- to postprogram: Early Interest in Geriatrics, Empathy/Compassion, Attitudes toward Geriatrics Careers, and Ageism.

The only significant interaction found between change in COCOA scores and baseline student characteristics was in gender, $F(1,132) = 5.71$, $p = .018$, such that male students' COCOA scores improved following the program participation, thereby diminishing the gap between male and female students' postprogram scores (Table 3). Project type did not have a statistically significant moderating effect.

In all the analyses, no severe departure from normality was detected for any of the analyses (t scores from the t tests and regression models) as determined by Q-Q plots and formal statistical tests for univariate normal distribution. There was also no evidence of multicollinearity, as the VIF was less than 1.5 for all covariates in the regression model. To ensure valid inference, we performed asymptotic permutation tests in addition to the t scores from the t tests and regression models and found virtually identical p values. Thus, results from the original t scores and associated p values are reported for the t tests and regression models (Table 4).

Table 3. Pre- and Postprogram Carolina Opinions on Care of Older Adults (COCOA) scores by subscale (N = 134).

COCOA[a] Subscale (Range)	Preprogram Mean (SD)	Postprogram Mean (SD)	t- or F score (df)	p Value
Early Interest in Geriatrics (5–25)	14.1 (4.3)	15.6 (4.2)	−5.87 (150)	< .001
Empathy/Compassion (4–20)	16.2 (2.4)	16.8 (2.3)	−3.82 (152)	< .001
Attitudes toward Geriatrics Careers (8–40)	28.4 (4.9)	29.8 (5.6)	−3.96 (153)	< .001
Ageism (9–45)	32.3 (5.0)	33.2 (5.4)	−2.67 (147)	= .008
Clinical and Social Services for Older Adults (11–55)	43.8 (6.1)	44.2 (7.1)	−.87 (142)	= .384
Social Value of Older Adults (5–25)	19.9 (2.5)	20.2 (2.8)	−1.69 (150)	= .093
COCOA Total (Range)				
Female COCOA Total (42–210)	156.2 (17.2)	158.9 (21.1)	5.71 (1, 132)	= .018
Male COCOA Total (42–210)	150.5 (17.9)	159.4 (17.9)		
COCOA total (42–210)	153.6 (17.7)	159.1 (19.6)	−4.22 (133)	< .001

Note. [a]COCOA Total score range = 42 – 210; COCOA items 1, 5, 7, 8, 9, 11, 12, 13, 18, 24, 25, 26, 27, 29, 30, 32, 33, 34, 36, 37, 39, 40, and 42 are reverse-scored.

Table 4. Linear regression model coefficients.

	Estimate (beta weight)	Standard Error	t Value	p Value
	Reduced (Trimmed) Model with Backward Elimination			
Intercept	2.70	1.81	1.50	.137
Male	6.51	2.70	2.42	.017
	Full (Initial) Model			
Intercept	5.42	4.32	1.25	.212
Male	6.15	2.74	2.24	.026
White	−3.34	2.88	−1.16	.249
MSTAR Program	−0.78	2.80	−0.28	.782
Top-20 medical school enrollment	1.60	2.74	0.58	.560
Clinical project type	−1.55	3.78	−0.41	.682
Translational project type	−4.30	4.80	−0.90	.371

Note. MSTAR = Medical Student Training in Aging Research
The baseline category for project type is basic project type.

Discussion

Our findings suggest that short-term research training programs focused on aging had a positive impact on medical students' attitudes toward older adults, especially in early interest in geriatrics, attitudes toward geriatrics careers, empathy and compassion toward older adults, and a reduction in ageism. These gains were made through mentored research training rather than a regular clinical rotation or an intervention explicitly focused on changing attitudes toward aging. There was a time by gender interaction, such that male medical students started out with worse attitudes than female student, but had a greater improvement, thereby exhibiting similar attitudes as females by the program's end.

This is, to our knowledge, the first study to indicate that aging-focused short-term research training can improve attitudes toward aging. There were multiple components within these programs that might have led to improved attitudes, including (1) exposure to aging-related research, and in some cases, research on successful aging (i.e., studies focusing on greater well-being among older adults); (2) participation in didactics on successful aging; (3) role modeling of mentors and program staff who had a strong interest in geriatrics, and exhibited optimism for improvement in health and well-being of older adults; (4) geriatric clinical experience, although limited, that offered some personal exposure to older adults; and (5) administration of the programs by a center with a focus on healthy aging. A recent review of interventions to elicit positive attitude change toward older adults among physicians and medical students found that interventions with an empathy-building component, such as mentoring, informal contact with older adults, or an aging simulation game appeared to be effective in changing attitudes (Samra, Griffiths, Cox, Conroy, & Knight, 2013). The MSTAR and M-STREAM programs incorporated mentoring and contact with older adults along with an emphasis on successful trajectories of aging. The COCOA subscales of early interest in geriatrics, empathy/ compassion, attitudes toward geriatrics careers, and ageism showed improvement following the programs, but clinical and social services for older adults, and social value of older adults did not. The MSTAR and M-STREAM programs offered very limited clinical and community exposure, and this may explain why these two domains did not improve.

Our findings of gender differences in attitudes toward aging are consistent with other studies reporting that female medical students generally have more positive attitudes toward seniors than their male counterparts (Fitzgerald et al., 2003; Hollar et al., 2011; Holtzman, Beck, & Ettinger, 1981; Reuben et al., 1995; Ruiz et al., 2015). In this study, male students demonstrated greater overall improvement in attitudes than female students, a finding that has also been reported in previous studies testing the effect of geriatric educational training and clinical exposure interventions on attitudes toward older adults (Hughes et al., 2008; Warren, Painter, & Rudisill, 1983). A likely explanation is that because females had high attitude scores preprogram, there was a ceiling effect for females, whereas male students had lower baseline scores, allowing room for improvement.

The finding of better attitudes toward aging among MSTAR compared to M-STREAM students at baseline might be due to self-selection bias. The MSTAR program focused on aging in a broad sense, whereas the M-STREAM focused on mental health and aging, perhaps drawing applicants with different views on aging in the context of health. It is not clear why students who undertook translational projects had higher COCOA scores than those undertaking clinical projects, or why students from top-20 medical schools demonstrated worse attitudes toward older adults. Possibly, more competitive medical schools need to pay greater attention to this area in their training curriculum.

There are several limitations to this study. It did not include a control group. The sample consisted of only first-year medical students from the United States, and therefore, the results may not generalize to other groups. Moreover, ours was a select group of medical students with expressed interest in aging, evidenced by their higher scores on COCOA compared to the scores reported among medical students in prior studies (Biese et al., 2011; Hollar et al., 2011), and therefore, these results may not represent all first-year medical students. It is not known whether gains in attitudes would persist at later time-points (e.g., at the end of medical school). Also, as our programs consisted of multiple components, we cannot be sure which particular components were responsible for changes in student attitudes. Finally, students who completed only the baseline COCOA assessment might have not exhibited the same level of improvement in attitudes as students who completed both sets of the measure.

Nonetheless, short-term aging-focused research training programs may be able to successfully foster positive attitudes toward seniors among medical students and, potentially, lead to larger numbers of physicians who decide to pursue a geriatrics (research) career. It is notable that the MSTAR and M-STREAM programs were associated with an increase in positive attitudes toward aging among the students who had already demonstrated an interest in geriatrics through their participation. Future directions for this work will include following-up with past trainees to track how many train for a career in geriatrics (Barron et al., 2015), incorporating clinical and community exposure into the programs, and including measures of implicit bias (Ruiz et al., 2015) to determine whether positive gains in self-report attitudes are reflected in the implicit attitudes of medical students toward seniors.

Acknowledgments

We want to thank Rebecca E. Daly for her invaluable help in data management.

Funding

Supported, in part, by: the National Institute on Aging T35 grant AG26757, the National Institutes of Health grant T35 AG026757/AG/NIA, the American Federation for Aging Research, the John A. Hartford Foundation, and the National Institutes of Health grant R25 MH071544/MH/NIMH, and by the Sam and Rose Stein Institute for Research on Aging at the University of California, San Diego.

References

American Geriatrics Society. (2011). Projection on future number of geriatricians in the United States. Retrieved from http://www.americangeriatrics.org/files/documents/gwps/Table%201_4.pdf

Atkinson, H. H., Lambros, A., Davis, B. R., Lawlor, J. S., Lovato, J., Sink, K. M., . . . Williamson, J. D. (2013). Teaching medical student geriatrics competencies in 1 week: An efficient model to teach and document selected competencies using clinical and community resources. *Journal of the American Geriatrics Society*, *61*(7), 1182–1187. doi:10.1111/jgs.12314

Barron, J. S., Bragg, E., Cayea, D., Durso, S. C., & Fedarko, N. S. (2015). The short-term and long-term impact of a brief aging research training program for medical students. *Gerontology & Geriatrics Education*, *36*(1), 96–106. doi:10.1080/02701960.2014.942036

Best Graduate Schools 2015. (2014). Washington, D.C.: U.S. News & World Report

Biese, K. J., Roberts, E., LaMantia, M., Zamora, Z., Shofer, F. S., Snyder, G., . . . Busby-Whitehead, J. (2011). Effect of a geriatric curriculum on emergency medicine resident attitudes, knowledge, and decision-making. *Academic Emergency Medicine : Official Journal of the Society for Academic Emergency Medicine*, *18*(Suppl 2), S92–96. doi:10.1111/j.1553-2712.2011.01170.x

Black, M. L., Curran, M. C., Golshan, S., Daly, R., Depp, C., Kelly, C., & Jeste, D. V. (2013). Summer research training for medical students: Impact on research self-efficacy. *Clinical and Translational Science*, *6*(6), 487–489. doi:10.1111/cts.12062

Center for Workforce Studies at the Association of American Medical Colleges. (2012). Physician specialty data book. Retrieved from https://members.aamc.org/eweb/upload/2012%20Physician%20Specialty%20Data%20Book.pdf

Committee on the Future Health Care Workforce for Older Americans Board on Health Care Services, Institute of Medicine. (2008). Retooling for an aging America: Building the health care workforce. Washington, D.C.: The National Academies Press Retrieved from http://www.iom.edu/Reports/2008/Retooling-for-an-Aging-America-Building-the-Health-Care-Workforce.aspx

Corwin, S. J., Frahm, K., Ochs, L. A., Rheaume, C. E., Roberts, E., & Eleazer, G. P. (2006). Medical student and senior participants' perceptions of a mentoring program designed to enhance geriatric medical education. *Gerontology & Geriatrics Education*, *26*(3), 47–65. doi:10.1300/J021v26n03_04

Dumbauld, J., Black, M., Depp, C. A., Daly, R., Curran, M. A., Winegarden, B., & Jeste, D. V. (2014). Association of learning styles with research self-efficacy: Study of short-term research training program for medical students. *Clinical and Translational Science*, *7*(6), 489–492. doi:10.1111/cts.12197

Duthie, E. H., Donnelly, M. B., & Kirsling, R. A. (1987). Fourth-year students' preference for geriatrics as a career. *Journal of Medical Education*, *62*(6), 511–514.

Effron, B., & Tibshirani, R. J. (1993). *An introduction to the bootstrap*. Boca Raton, FL: Chapman & Hall.

Fitzgerald, J. T., Wray, L. A., Halter, J. B., Williams, B. C., & Supiano, M. A. (2003). Relating medical students' knowledge, attitudes, and experience to an interest in geriatric medicine. *Gerontologist*, *43*(6), 849–855. doi:10.1093/geront/43.6.849

Hollar, D., Roberts, E., & Busby-Whitehead, J. (2011). COCOA: A new validated instrument to assess medical students' attitudes towards older adults. *Educational Gerontology*, *37*(3), 193–209. doi:10.1080/03601277.2010.532063

Holtzman, J. M., Beck, J. D., & Ettinger, R. L. (1981). Cognitive knowledge and attitudes toward the aged of dental and medical students. *Educational Gerontology*, *6*(2/3), 195–207. doi:10.1080/0380127810060210

Hughes, N. J., Soiza, R. L., Chua, M., Hoyle, G. E., MacDonald, A., Primrose, W. R., & Gwyn Seymour, D. (2008). Medical student attitudes toward older people and willingness to consider a career in geriatric medicine. *Journal of the American Geriatrics Society*, *56*(2), 334–338. doi:10.1111/j.1532-5415.2007.01552.x

Jeste, D. V., Halpain, M. C., Trinidad, G. I., Reichstadt, J. L., & Lebowitz, B. D. (2007). UCSD's short-term research training programs for trainees at different levels of career development. *Academic Psychiatry*, *31*(2), 160–167. doi:10.1176/appi.ap.31.2.160

Kearney, N., Miller, M., Paul, J., & Smith, K. (2000). Oncology healthcare professionals' attitudes toward elderly people. *Annals of Oncology : Official Journal of the European Society for Medical Oncology / ESMO, 11*(5), 599–601. doi:10.1023/A:1008327129699

Laks, J., Wilson, L. A., Khandelwal, C., Footman, E., Jamison, M., & Roberts, E. (2016). Service-Learning in Communities of Elders (SLICE): Development and evaluation of an introductory geriatrics course for medical students. *Teaching and Learning in Medicine, 28*(2), 210–218. doi:10.1080/10401334.2016.1146602

Madan, A. K., Aliabadi-Wahle, S., & Beech, D. J. (2001). Age bias: A cause of underutilization of breast conservation treatment. *Journal of Cancer Education : the Official Journal of the American Association for Cancer Education, 16*(1), 29–32. doi:10.1080/08858190109528720

Meisner, B. A. (2012). Physicians' attitudes toward aging, the aged, and the provision of geriatric care: A systematic narrative review. *Critical Public Health, 22*(1), 61–72. doi:10.1080/09581596.2010.539592

Federal Interagency Forum on Aging-Related Statistics. (2016). *Older Americans* 2016: *Key indicators of well-being*. Retrieved from https://agingstats.gov/docs/LatestReport/Older-Americans-2016-Key-Indicators-of-WellBeing.pdf

Perrotta, P., Perkins, D., Schimpfhauser, F., & Calkins, E. (1981). Medical student attitudes toward geriatric medicine and patients. *Journal of Medical Education, 56*(6), 478–483.

Reuben, D. B., Fullerton, J. T., Tschann, J. M., & Croughan-Minihane, M. (1995). Attitudes of beginning medical students toward older persons: A five-campus study. The university of california academic geriatric resource program student survey research group. *Journal of the American Geriatrics Society, 43*(12), 1430–1436. doi:10.1111/j.1532-5415.1995.tb06626.x

Ruiz, J. G., Andrade, A. D., Anam, R., Taldone, S., Karanam, C., Hogue, C., & Mintzer, M. J. (2015). Group-based differences in anti-aging bias among medical students. *Gerontology & Geriatrics Education, 36*(1), 58–78. doi:10.1080/02701960.2014.966904

Samra, R., Griffiths, A., Cox, T., Conroy, S., & Knight, A. (2013). Changes in medical student and doctor attitudes toward older adults after an intervention: A systematic review. *Journal of the American Geriatrics Society, 61*(7), 1188–1196. doi:10.1111/jgs.12312

Smith, B. D., Haffty, B. G., Wilson, L. D., Smith, G. L., Patel, A. N., & Buchholz, T. A. (2010). The future of radiation oncology in the United States from 2010 to 2020: Will supply keep pace with demand? *Journal of Clinical Oncology : Official Journal of the American Society of Clinical Oncology, 28*(35), 5160–5165. doi:10.1200/jco.2010.31.2520

Tang, W., He, H., & Xin M., T. (2012). *Applied categorical and count data analysis.* Boca Raton, FL: CRC Press.

Thorson, J. A., & Powell, F. C. (1991). Medical students' attitudes towards ageing and death: A cross-sequential study. *Medical Education, 25*(1), 32–37. doi:10.1111/j.1365-2923.1991.tb00023.x

Varkey, P., Chutka, D. S., & Lesnick, T. G. (2006). The Aging Game: Improving medical students' attitudes toward caring for the elderly. *Journal of the American Medical Directors Association, 7*(4), 224–229. doi:10.1016/j.jamda.2005.07.009

Voogt, S. J., Mickus, M., Santiago, O., & Herman, S. E. (2008). Attitudes, experiences, and interest in geriatrics of first-year allopathic and osteopathic medical students. *Journal of the American Geriatrics Society, 56*(2), 339–344. doi:10.1111/j.1532-5415.2007.01541.x

Warren, D. L., Painter, A., & Rudisill, J. (1983). Effects of geriatric education on the attitudes of medical students. *Journal of the American Geriatrics Society, 31*(7), 435–438. doi:10.1111/j.1532-5415.1983.tb03720.x

Warshaw, G., & Bragg, E. (2008). *Projection on future number of geriatric psychiatrists in the United States.* Retrieved from http://www.americangeriatrics.org/files/documents/gwps/Table%201_29.pdf

Wilkinson, T. J., Gower, S., & Sainsbury, R. (2002). The earlier, the better: The effect of early community contact on the attitudes of medical students to older people. *Medical Education, 36*(6), 540–542. doi:10.1046/j.1365-2923.2002.01226.x

Wilson, J. F., & Hafferty, F. W. (1980). Changes in attitudes toward the elderly one year after a seminar on aging and health. *Journal of Medical Education, 55*(12), 993–999.

Medical students' reflections of a posthospital discharge patient visit

Linda Pang, Reena Karani, and Sara M. Bradley

ABSTRACT

Transitions of care is an important part of patient safety that is not often taught in medical schools. As part of a curriculum for patient safety and transitions of care, third-year medical students followed patients they cared for during their inpatient rotations on a posthospital discharge visit. Students answered reflection questions on these visits, which were reviewed at a group debriefing session. The written reflections and oral debriefings were analyzed qualitatively to identify what medical students were able to learn from a posthospital discharge visit. Of the students who visited patients, 265 participated in the debriefing sessions, and their responses were grouped into 7 domains and 33 themes. Students commented most often on the importance of family and caregivers who provided support for the patient after hospitalization. They identified problems specific to the discharge process and factors that helped or hindered transitions, noted new experiences visiting postacute care facilities, and also developed solutions to improve transitions. Postdischarge visits combined with brief reflection writing and debriefing allowed students to better understand difficulties that can be faced in care transitions.

Background

Patients often undergo transitions from one care setting to another. Poor coordination between care teams during these times can compromise the quality of patient care, resulting in adverse outcomes such as medication errors and avoidable hospital readmissions. Research shows that up to 20% of hospitalized patients experience an adverse event within 3 weeks of discharge and that up to one third of these events could have been prevented (Coleman, 2003). Avoiding posthospital discharge adverse events is especially important in geriatric care because older adults constitute 13% of the U.S. population but 37% of all patients hospitalized for acute-care needs (Hall, DeFrances, Williams, Golosinskiy, & Schwartzman, 2010). Older adults also have longer hospital stays, more transitions of care after hospitalization, and a higher risk of readmission (Coleman, Min, Chomiak, & Kramer, 2004; Ma, Coleman, Fish, Lin, & Kramer, 2004; Podrazik & Whelan, 2008).

Organizations like the Accreditation Council for Graduate Medical Education (2015) and the Association of American Medical Colleges (2014) have increasingly encouraged incorporating patient safety and transitions-of-care curricula into medical education. Communicating key components of a safe discharge plan is also part of the minimum geriatric competencies for medical students as determined by a systematic multimethod consensus process in 2007 (Leipzig et al., 2009). However, the patient safety and quality improvement curricula described in the medical education literature focus more on the education of residents than on medical students, with classroom-based didactic sessions being the most common instructional method (Buchanan & Besdine, 2011; Wong, Etchells, Kuper, Levinson, & Shojania, 2010). Other teaching methods used include reflective learning, experiential learning, and interdisciplinary training (Block, Morgan-Gouveia, Levine, & Cayea, 2014; Lai, Nye, Bookwalter, Kwan, & Hauer, 2008; McNabney, Willging, Fried, & Durso, 2009). Transitions-of-care curricula incorporating post-hospital discharge patient visits have been shown to improve medical students' knowledge, attitudes, and confidence in their skills regarding transitions of care and discharge planning (Bray-Hall, Schmidt, & Aagaard, 2010; Lai et al., 2008; Ouchida, LoFaso, Capello, Ramsaroop, & Reid, 2009).

We previously published an evaluation of a patient safety and transitions-of-care curriculum for 3rd-year medical students. This curriculum was part of a formal Integrated Internal Medicine-Geriatrics Clerkship. Quantitative analysis of pre- and postintervention assessments showed that students' knowledge of and confidence about patient safety and other key aspects of transitions of care substantially improved as a result of the curriculum (Bradley, Chang, Fallar, & Karani, 2015). An important component of that curriculum was a posthospital discharge visit to patients the students had cared for in the hospital, followed by opportunities for students to reflect and debrief about the patient visits. Although prior studies mainly focused on the quantitative assessment of patient safety and transitions-of-care curriculum, the objective of the present study was to understand what 3rd-year medical students learned from posthospital discharge visits through analysis of qualitative data collected from the students' written reflections and oral debriefing sessions (Bray-Hall et al., 2010; Lai et al., 2008).

Method

Study setting and data collection

Third-year medical students ($N = 277$) took part in a patient safety and transitions of care curriculum between 2012 and 2014. This curriculum was part of a mandatory 12-week Integrated Internal Medicine-Geriatrics Clerkship. The clerkship was divided into three blocks: 4 weeks of inpatient medicine at a quaternary hospital, 4 weeks of inpatient medicine at a community hospital, and 4 weeks of geriatric medicine. The geriatric medicine block included 2 weeks in a hospital-based ambulatory geriatrics practice, 1 week of palliative medicine, and 1 week with a house-call program providing care to homebound elderly patients.

The patient safety and transitions of care curriculum included a series of interactive didactics spread throughout the clerkship. These lectures focused on patient safety, health literacy, transitions of care, and discharge planning. Students also participated in posthospital discharge visits. During their 4 weeks of inpatient medicine at the quaternary hospital, students were asked to identify a patient they had cared for to visit after discharge. Students were encouraged to choose patients older than age 65. Later, while the students were participating in the geriatric medicine portion of the clerkship, they went in pairs to visit their patients at home or in an assisted living facility, rehabilitation center, or nursing home. Almost one half (48%) of students visited their own patients whereas the remainder visited their partner's patient. The study was registered with the Grants and Contracts Office of Icahn School of Medicine at Mount Sinai and determined exempt from Institutional Review Board review.

To guide their patient visits, the students were given a template of questions that focused on factors known to be important during care transitions (Coleman, 2003; Snow et al., 2009). The questions aimed to ascertain whether patients had copies of their discharge instructions; whether patients understood the reason for their hospitalization; whether patients understood their new medications or medication changes; whether patients had been able to obtain their medications; whether patients were aware of their follow-up appointments, tests, and services; the state of the patients' health since discharge; whether patients were aware of the warning signs of adverse events; and whether patients knew how to contact their providers in the case of problems after discharge. In some cases, caregivers were also present, and students included them in the posthospital discharge visit discussions.

After the visit, students were asked to write answers to the following reflective questions: "How did the visit go for you?" "How was the dynamic with the patient different from when they were in the hospital?" "Was there anything that surprised you about the visit, such as the patient's understanding, or lack of it, of their hospitalization or the patient's home environment?" and "Do you think this experience will affect how you communicate with patients at discharge in the future? If yes, in what way?" Our questions were open ended to give students the opportunity a wide variety of topics they felt important in their posthospital discharge visits. The visits and the students' written answers to the reflective questions were reviewed at 1-hour group debriefing sessions held at the end of each month. The debriefing sessions were attended by 12 to 13 students who had recently completed their geriatrics blocks. The sessions were led by the clerkship directors. All participants gave permission to be recorded. A total of 11 debriefing sessions were recorded and analyzed.

Data analysis

Debriefing sessions conducted from July 2012 to June 2014 were audio-recorded and transcribed verbatim by a professional transcription service in a deidentified manner. The transcripts were analyzed using the constant comparative method associated with grounded theory (Strauss & Corbin, 1990). Two coders (LP, SB) independently analyzed transcripts from the first year of the study to identify preliminary codes. The coders then met to group the preliminary codes into themes. The coders then independently recoded the year 1 transcripts and coded the year 2 transcripts using the identified themes. Finally, they met to check for intercoder agreement; disputes were resolved by discussion and joint review of transcript passages.

Several steps were taken to verify the results and ensure their trustworthiness. First, the two coders performed the initial coding independently. After coding, the resulting themes were validated by triangulation, that is, by comparing students' written responses to the reflective questions with their verbal responses from the debriefing sessions. Additionally, member checking was used to assess trustworthiness; some of the student participants were asked to review the themes for their effectiveness in capturing their perspectives. Quotations that the researchers judged to be representative of the responses for each theme were selected for inclusion in this paper. Minor edits for clarity and grammar were made to the quotations. A total of 277 students completed the clerkship during the study period. Of these, 265 (96%) students participated in the debriefing sessions.

Results

Students contributed 388 individual comments during the debriefing sessions, which were grouped into 33 themes. These themes were then organized into seven domains: (1) problems specific to discharge itself, (2) factors associated with safe or unsafe transitions, (3) students' suggested solutions to problems in transitions of care, (4) patients' experience in the community, (5) students' impressions of skilled nursing facilities, (6) problems during hospitalization, and (7) potentially unavoidable readmissions. More than 50% of the comments were related to the problems specific to discharge itself and factors associated with safe or unsafe transitions. Table 1 shows the distribution of comments by domain and theme.

Problems specific to discharge

This domain, which included comments related to communication during the discharge process, accounted for 27.6% of all comments (107/388). Seven themes fell under this domain:

Table 1. Domains and themes of medical students' reflections of patient visit.

Domains and Themes	No. of Comments (% total)
Problems specific to discharge	107 (27.6%)
Patients lacked understanding of reason for hospitalization	24
Medication errors	20
Problem with discharge summary	20
Lack of communication with outpatient caregivers and providers	13
Follow-up appointment errors	11
Use of emergency services	10
Discharge felt rushed	9
Factors associated with safe or unsafe transitions	93 (24.0%)
Family/caregiver support	34
Access to community services	15
Health literacy	13
Socioeconomic status	7
Language barrier	7
Insurance	6
Age was not a barrier	6
Cognitive impairment	5
Student solutions to problems in transitions of care	62 (16.0%)
Better patient education during hospital stay	27
Solutions specific to discharge summary	12
Solutions specific to medication reconciliation	8
Better communication with primary care provider	8
Education and involvement of caregiver	7
Patients' experience in the community	49 (12.6%)
Positive change in emotional and physical appearance	22
More functional	10
Change in power dynamic	9
Understand patient in larger social context	8
Impressions of skilled nursing facilities	37 (9.5%)
Similar to hospital environment	12
Isolating/depressing environment	9
First exposure for students to this type of facility	7
Family did not have discharge paperwork	4
Lack of patient's functional recovery	3
Difficulty communicating with staff	2
Problems during hospitalization	26 (6.7%)
Fragmented health care system	13
Constraints limiting team-patient relationship	8
Uncertainty in medicine	5
Potentially unavoidable readmissions	14 (3.6%)

(1) lack of patient knowledge about their reason for hospitalization, (2) medication errors, (3) discharge summary problems, (4) lack of communication with outpatient caregivers and/or providers, (5) follow-up appointment errors, (6) use of emergency services, and (7) rushed discharge. The most commonly cited theme in this domain (24/107) was lack of patient knowledge of their reason for hospitalization. Students spoke of patients who did not understand medical terminology, the severity of their illness, or all parts of their complicated hospital stay. After visiting a patient at a rehabilitation facility, one student commented,

> She didn't have a really good handle as to what COPD was. When we asked her what brought you to the hospital..., she didn't even know what to call it. She says, "I had an exacerbation. There's something in my lung," and I was like, "Do you mean a COPD exacerbation?" ... I think she thought of it almost as a mass or something.... How these things can fall through the crack even though she is very with it in the other parts of her life in terms of managing the difficult navigation of insurance and getting that.... Somehow despite—this lady, who's very smart and very bright, did not understand her disease. That was striking.

Another frequent theme of students' comments in this domain was medication errors (20/107). Students commented that miscommunication between care teams resulted in patients' being unsure of which instructions to follow. On their posthospital discharge visits, students noticed barriers preventing patients from getting their medications, such as the need for prior approval from insurance providers, the expense of medications, and patients' lack of knowledge about their discharge medication regimens. One student recounted:

> He thought he had the needle for the insulin pen, but when he went to the pharmacy, they didn't have it for him.... So they went home. They tried to manage his diabetes by not giving him fatty food, but the next day he was dizzy and then comes in again. So this time before he left the second time, we made sure that he physically had insulin syringes with him and needles.

Students also commonly cited problems with discharge summaries (20/107). For example, students described some summaries as "unreadable," "poorly formatted," and "containing too much information." When one student saw the discharge summary sent home with a patient, he was alarmed to find that it looked like a draft version and not the final summary. Another student commented:

> Reading through what the information was, I was really disappointed, because they attach five pages of generic warning symptoms that are completely worthless ... rather than the reason that you were in the hospital and what we did for you as the front and center.... Why can't we write a medically simplified one that somebody, who can take care of a patient or perhaps the patient themselves, can interpret, even if it's a couple of sentences?

Factors associated with safe or unsafe transitions

About one fourth (93/388) of the comments focused on factors associated with safe or unsafe transitions. These comments fell into eight themes: (1) family or caregiver support, (2) access to community services, (3) health literacy, (4) socioeconomic status, (5) language barriers, (6) insurance, (7) older age not seen as a barrier, and (8) cognitive impairment. Students most frequently commented on the importance of the caregivers who supported the patients. For example, several students spoke of home attendants who were more knowledgeable than the patients about the patients' illnesses and medications. They saw family members who coordinated complicated medication regimens or multiple appointments. Conversely, some students noted how lack of family involvement—for example, when a spouse was cognitively impaired—made the posthospital discharge transition more difficult. One student reflected:

> I was amazed by how involved and committed the family was to the patient's care. As the patient is immobile and on a ventilator, the patient's care is completely coordinated by her husband and daughters. It was stunning and inspiring how every member of the family was completely committed to making sure everything was being done correctly—from administering a complex medical regimen, to checking bi-daily blood sugars and blood pressure, to having one person sleep in the patient's room every night, to calling and coordinating visits from visiting nurse services, physical therapy, occupational therapy, and respiratory therapy. It was clear that taking care of a family member can be a tiring, full-time job.

Student solutions to problems with transitions of care

Sixteen percent (62/388) of the students' comments were suggestions for solutions to issues the students had noted in the discharge transition process. Five themes emerged in this domain: (1) better patient education during the hospital stay, (2) solutions specific to the discharge summary, (3) solutions specific to medication reconciliation, (4) better communication with the primary care provider, and (5) education and involvement of caregivers. Regarding the most common theme, better patient education (27/62 comments), students suggested using the teach-back method more often, breaking information into smaller chunks for daily teaching, and focusing on the kinds of potential discharge obstacles that often result in readmission. One student suggested:

> I was thinking it should be treated like a sign-out to the patient themselves when you discharge them.... "If this happens, this is what you should do." ... I think people do a wonderful job, but I don't think we use the same diligence that we do when handing over to the overnight team when we hand a patient's health back into their own hands.

Students also spoke about actions they had implemented during their inpatient rotations to improve their discharge summaries (12/62 comments). One student made a calendar of the patient's future appointments, and another translated the summary into the patient's primary language. Regarding medication reconciliation (8/62 comments), students felt it was necessary to explicitly discuss each discharge medication with patients. They noted a variety of reasons why patients did not take their medications at home, including concerns about side effects or not understanding the reason for the medications. A few students suggested strategizing with patients to determine methods for ensuring compliance, such as using a pill box, alarm, or alternative tactics such as rubber-banding medications bottles to group together to take at the same time.

Patients in the community

About 13% (49/388) of the comments pertained to students' observations of their patients outside of the hospital. Four themes emerged: (1) a positive change in emotional and physical appearance, (2) increased functional ability, (3) a change in the power dynamic between the patient and the health care team, and (4) the opportunity for students to understand patients in a larger social context. When students visited their patients at home, they found their patients to be happier and more confident than they had been in the hospital. One student noted:

> When we went to visit her, she was so excited and happy, and seemed so healthy, and just in her element at home, and there were kids running around, and it was a very joyous environment. It was very striking because in the hospital she was weak and in a really negative state.... When we were talking with her yesterday, she was embracing life and how she doesn't want to just sit in a corner. It was such a different mentality.

Students also reacted positively to seeing their patients in a different context than that of acute hospitalization and illness (8/49 comments). They described learning much more about their patients' social histories in the home environment and found that seeing patients in their home settings had a humanizing effect. One student reflected:

> Part of this three months has taught us all how to present really well, which means, social history is do they smoke, do they drink, and are they sexually active? That's not how patients define their own social history. So it was cool to see the transition of her from a very vulnerable place where she could hardly speak without panting to understand her as the center of her entire family. She was taking care of her mom and her grandkids and her grandkids' pets, and she's been in the same building since she was a kid and knows every drug dealer in that building, and they love her. What that said to me ... is her illness [was] taking a toll on an entire microcommunity and they all needed her.

Students' impressions of skilled nursing facilities

Some students were able to visit their patients at skilled nursing facilities, either in rehabilitation units or in long-term care. About 10% (37/388) of the students' comments were related to their impressions of these facilities. We divided the comments into six themes: (1) the similarity to a hospital environment, (2) the isolating or depressing environment, (3) students' first exposure to this type of facility, (4) family members not provided with discharge paperwork, (5) patients' lack of functional recovery at the facility, and (6) difficulties in communication with staff at the facilities. Students noted they could not find nursing or other staff at the facility to ask questions or pass on patient requests. The most frequent theme in this domain was the noted similarity to the hospital (12/37). One student remarked:

> It was a pretty eye-opening experience, the capacity the nursing home has. It looks kind of like a mini-ward.... The rooms each look like hospital bedrooms, and the nursing staff all knew the patients pretty well, but were so unbelievably overwhelmed.

Problems during hospitalization

Students noted that for some patients, problems during hospitalization negatively affected a patient's transition of care. This domain accounted for about 7% of all comments (26/388). Three themes fell under this domain: (1) a fragmented health care system, (2) constraints limiting the team–patient relationship, and (3) uncertainty in medicine. Sometimes, despite hospitalization, patients did not get the specific answers they were seeking for their problems and left still with uncertainty. Students spoke about difficulties receiving time-sensitive information for patients to continue effective hospital care. With regards to a fragmented health care system, one student recounted:

I try to get records for this lady who has biliary tract cancer so I wanted to get the GI consult notes. It literally took me three days calling. I still didn't get it. They sent me everything except for the thing I needed. It's just amazing. She has cancer that is terminal, but they can't give me 15 days of paper [progress notes]. And it shows how insanely difficult it is to operate within different systems. This patient's [primary care provider] wasn't at [our hospital] and that was a huge deal. It really shows the benefit of having all their care in one system. But obviously everybody doesn't have that option.

Potentially unavoidable readmissions

This domain accounted for 3.6% of all comments (14/388). Students noted that many patients in the quaternary hospital setting were quite ill or had extensive and complicated medical problems. Some of these patients were frequently readmitted despite the care teams' best attempts to coordinate care transitions.

Discussion

This study demonstrated that posthospital discharge patient visits allowed students to better understand difficulties that can be faced in care transitions. The medical students in this study identified patient safety problems specific to the discharge process that have also been identified in previous studies, such as a lack of knowledge about the reasons for hospitalization and medication errors (Block et al., 2014). The students also identified several key factors, such as community support services and health literacy, as components contributing to safer transitions of care, and they recommended solutions, such as enhanced patient education and clearer discharge summaries, to improve patient care after hospitalization. The issues identified are consistent with problems noted in the patient safety literature (Snow et al., 2009). Moreover, our students provided compelling stories of lessons learned about patient safety that they could not have realized without a posthospital discharge visit. They were very moved by the degree of caregiver support at home, were engaged in new experiences in postacute care, and saw the continued positive transformation of patients who had been discharged back to their communities.

In this study, visiting patients outside of the hospital allowed medical students to grasp the importance of family and caregiver support in safe transitions of care. They were often surprised at the extent to which caregivers needed to be involved in these situations. The beneficial relationships of patients and those who care for them on a routine basis are often invisible in an inpatient setting, where the focus tends to be on stabilization of an acute medical condition. There is also lack of formal literature teaching medical students to understand the role caregivers play in supporting older adults. As recognition of the role of paid and unpaid caregivers grows, it will be imperative for medical students to understand the importance of involving older patients' caregivers in the discharge process (Germain et al., 2016; Kasper, Freedman, Spillman, & Wolff, 2015). We propose that the kind of curriculum described here may help to deepen discussions of this underrecognized issue.

The posthospital discharge visit could serve as a platform for increasing medical students' exposure to postacute care settings. Nationally, 22% of all hospital discharges are to a postacute care setting (Tian, 2016). However, the nursing home setting is often overlooked in medical education with only 32% of medical students having field experience in nursing home care in a recent AAMC 2016 Medical School Graduation Questionnaire . In our program, the posthospital discharge visit allowed students to visit skilled nursing facilities that are often neglected in internal medicine curricula. For some students, this was the first experience with nursing home care. The nursing home can be a useful site in which students can practice skills such as medical interviewing and collaborating in an interprofessional environment (Huls, De Rooij, Diepstraten, Koopmans, & Helmich, 2015). However, in our curriculum, which involved a single visit without guidance by staff, students often had negative experiences. Students reported perceiving that the care was isolating and having difficulty communicating with staff. Having an educational champion at these sites would likely improve students' experiences. Seeing patients in skilled nursing facilities and under-standing the benefits and limits of these settings can help medical students to learn to make shared decisions with patients about expectations for posthospital care.

Students who visited their patients at home often gave rich detail about their patients' changes after discharge back into their communities. Students were often surprised by the positive changes in the dynamics, functioning, and well-being of their patients at home. These dramatic differences could not have been appreciated without the posthospital discharge visit. The students learned that when transitions of care go well, even patients who are seriously ill can improve outside of the inpatient setting. Furthermore, seeing patients in their own homes was enriching for students; they learned to see patients as more than just their medical illnesses, as participants in the broader social contexts of their communities.

During the debriefings, we noted that students often worked with patients to devise creative solutions to the problems they encountered. Some of their solutions, such as keeping an appointment calendar, communicating with outside providers, and providing language-specific material, are consistent with actions recommended by nationwide groups to reduce rehospitalizations (Hansen, Young, Hinami, Leung, & Williams, 2011; Jack et al., 2009). Seeing the outcomes of poor transitions during their posthospital discharge visits led students to apply their own experiences to initiate simple yet effective solutions. This could serve as a springboard from which students could lead larger quality improvement projects within their educational communities.

This study had some limitations. We studied a single urban medical center, which may limit the generalizability of our results. Without a control group, we were unable to determine whether the themes that emerged in students' reflections may have been drawn from components of the curriculum that were not specific to the posthospital discharge patient visit, reflection writing, and debriefing session. However, we noted that several of the identified themes were specific to the students' seeing their patients outside of the hospital environment, suggesting that this component of the curriculum did provide a pedagogical benefit. Because the debriefing transcripts were deidentified, we were unable to tell if all students participated equally. For instance, some students were not able to visit their own patients and, as a result, may not have shared as much as students who visited their own patients did. To account for students who may have preferred solo written reflection to group oral debriefing, we triangulated themes found in the debriefing session transcripts with students' written responses to the reflection questions; we did not find any themes that were specific to the written reflections. This study was also unable to fully assess whether the comments indicate an attitudinal change on the part of the medical students or whether their newly acquired knowledge will persist and guide their clinical experience during residency training.

In our next steps, we hope to allow every medical student to see a patient they cared for in the hospital in a posthospital discharge visit. We believe allowing students to follow their own patient may have a stronger impact in their experiential learning process. Medical students will be asked to identify three potential patients in their inpatient clerkship to visit on a posthospital discharge. We also hope to use the affiliate sites of our expanded medical center in order to provide a greater opportunity for students to visit their own patients. As we learned through the debriefing sessions that the posthospital discharge visit was a useful time for students to be exposed to rehabilitation units and long-term care facilities, we will change our curriculum to enhance this exposure. Students will be asked to focus their posthospital discharge visits on patients being discharged to rehabilitation units and long-term care facilities with which our institution has already formed an educational collaboration. We hope to use this opportunity to enrich our curriculum and teach about interdisciplinary care as this frail population undergoes multiple transitions of care. To improve patient care and medical student discharge education, we will modify our discharge planning didactic session to include health literacy and discharge education tools such as the teach-back method. We want to encourage our medical students to be actively involved in the discharge process by having them discuss medication reconciliation using discharge education tools learned. This will also enhance the medical students' education by allowing them to rapidly re-evaluate their own skillset when following up with the patients they have taught on the posthospital discharge visit.

As our nation experiences a growth in the population of older adults, who are more likely to be hospitalized and to experience adverse events associated with hospitalization, future health care providers need training about patient safety and transitions of care. In conclusion, a posthospital discharge patient visit combined with written reflection and a debriefing exercise allowed our medical students to identify problems associated with safe transitions of care and to develop solutions to these problems. Including posthospital discharge visits in geriatrics curricula is a feasible way to complement and highlight other forms of pedagogy on these important topics.

Acknowledgments

Preliminary results were presented at the Geriatric Education Paper Session, American Geriatrics Society Annual Meeting, Long Beach, CA, May 19, 2016.

References

Accreditation Council for Graduate Medical Education and American Board of Internal Medicine. (2015). *The internal medicine residency milestones project.* Retrieved from http://www.acgme.org/portals/0/pdfs/milestones/internalmedicinemilestones.pdf

Association of American Medical Colleges. (2014). *Core entrustable professional activities for entering residency: Curriculum developers' guide.* Retrieved from http://members.aamc.org/eweb/upload/Core%20EPA%20Curriculum%20Dev%20Guide.pdf

Association of American Medical Colleges. (2016). *Medical school graduation questionnaire: 2016 all schools summary report.* Retrieved from http://www.aamc.org/download/474412/data/2016gqallschoolssummaryreport.pdf

Block, L., Morgan-Gouveia, M., Levine, R. B., & Cayea, D. (2014). We could have done a better job: A qualitative study of medical student reflections on safe hospital discharge. *Journal of the American Geriatrics Society, 62*(6), 1147–1154. doi:10.1111/jgs.12783

Bradley, S. M., Chang, D., Fallar, R., & Karani, R. (2015). A patient safety and transitions of care curriculum for third-year medical students. *Gerontology & Geriatrics Education, 36*(1), 45–57. doi:10.1080/02701960.2014.966903

Bray-Hall, S., Schmidt, K., & Aagaard, E. (2010). Toward safe hospital discharge: A transitions in care curriculum for medical students. *Journal of General Internal Medicine, 25*(8), 878–881. doi:10.1007/s11606-010-1364-3

Buchanan, I. M., & Besdine, R. W. (2011). A systematic review of curricular interventions teaching transitional care to physicians-in-training and physicians. *Academic Medicine : Journal of the Association of American Medical Colleges, 86*(5), 628–639. doi:10.1097/ACM.0b013e318212e36c

Coleman, E. A. (2003). Falling through the cracks: Challenges and opportunities for improving transitional care for persons with continuous complex care needs. *Journal of the American Geriatrics Society, 51*(4), 549–555. doi:10.1046/j.1532-5415.2003.51185.x

Coleman, E. A., Min, S. J., Chomiak, A., & Kramer, A. M. (2004). Posthospital care transitions: patterns, complications, and risk identification. Health Serv Res, 39(5),1449–1465. doi:10.1111/j.1475-6773.2004.00298.x

Germain, V., Dabakuyo-Yonli, T. S., Marilier, S., Putot, A., Bengrine-Lefevre, L., Arveux, P., & Quipourt, V. (2016). Management of elderly patients suffering from cancer: Assessment of perceived burden and of quality of life of primary caregivers. *Journal of Geriatric Oncology* doi:10.1016/j.jgo.2016.12.001.

Hall, M. J., DeFrances, C. J., Williams, S. N., Golosinskiy, A., & Schwartzman, A. (2010). National hospital discharge survey: 2007 summary. *National Health Statistics Reports, 24*(29), 1–20.

Hansen, L. O., Young, R. S., Hinami, K., Leung, A., & Williams, M. V. (2011). Interventions to reduce 30-day rehospitalization: A systematic review. *Annals of Internal Medicine, 155*(8), 520–528. doi:10.7326/0003-4819-155-8-201110180-00008

Huls, M., De Rooij, S. E., Diepstraten, A., Koopmans, R., & Helmich, E. (2015). Learning to care for older patients: Hospitals and nursing homes as learning environments. *Medical Education, 49*(3), 332–339. doi:10.1111/medu.12646

Jack, B. W., Chetty, V. K., Anthony, D., Greenwald, J. L., Sanchez, G. M., Johnson, A. E., & Culpepper, L. (2009). A reengineered hospital discharge program to decrease rehospitalization: A randomized trial. *Annals of Internal Medicine, 150*(3), 178–187. doi:10.7326/0003-4819-150-3-200902030-00007

Kasper, J. D., Freedman, V. A., Spillman, B. C., & Wolff, J. L. (2015). The disproportionate impact of dementia on family and unpaid caregiving to older adults. *Health Affairs (Project Hope), 34*(10), 1642–1649. doi:10.1377/hlthaff.2015.0536

Lai, C. J., Nye, H. E., Bookwalter, T., Kwan, A., & Hauer, K. E. (2008). Postdischarge follow-up visits for medical and pharmacy students on an inpatient medicine clerkship. *Journal of Hospital Medicine : An Official Publication of the Society of Hospital Medicine, 3*(1), 20–27. doi:10.1002/jhm.264

Leipzig, R. M., Granville, L., Simpson, D., Anderson, M. B., Sauvigne, K., & Soriano, R. P. (2009). Keeping granny safe on July 1: A consensus on minimum geriatrics competencies for graduating medical students. *Academic Medicine : Journal of the Association of American Medical Colleges, 84*(5), 604–610. doi:10.1097/ACM.0b013e31819fab70

Ma, E., Coleman, E. A., Fish, R., Lin, M., & Kramer, A. M. (2004). Quantifying posthospital care transitions in older patients. J Am Med Dir Assoc, 5(2),71–74. doi:10.1097/01.jam.0000110658.01514.f7

McNabney, M. K., Willging, P. R., Fried, L. P., & Durso, S. C. (2009). The "continuum of care" for older adults: Design and evaluation of an educational series. *Journal of the American Geriatrics Society, 57*(6), 1088–1095. doi:10.1111/j.1532-5415.2009.02275.x

Ouchida, K., LoFaso, V. M., Capello, C. F., Ramsaroop, S., & Reid, M. C. (2009). Fast forward rounds: An effective method for teaching medical students to transition patients safely across care settings. *Journal of the American Geriatrics Society*, *57*(5), 910–917. doi:10.1111/j.1532-5415.2009.02203.x

Podrazik, P. M., & Whelan, C. T. (2008). Acute hospital care for the elderly patient: its impact on clinical and hospital systems of care. Med Clin North Am, 92(2),387–406, ix.

Snow, V., Beck, D., Budnitz, T., Miller, D. C., Potter, J., Wears, R. L., ... Williams, M. V. (2009). Transitions of care consensus policy statement American College of Physicians-Society of General Internal Medicine-Society of Hospital Medicine-American Geriatrics Society-American College of Emergency Physicians-Society of Academic Emergency Medicine. *Journal of General Internal Medicine*, *24*(8), 971–976. doi:10.1007/s11606-009-0969-x

Strauss A, Corbin JM. Basics of Qualitative Research: Grounded Theory Procedures and Techniques. Thousand Oaks, Calif: Sage Publications; 1990.

Tian W. (AHRQ). An All-Payer View of Hospital Discharge to Postacute Care, 2013. HCUP Statistical Brief #205. May 2016. Agency for Healthcare Research and Quality, Rockville, MD. http://www.hcup-us.ahrq.gov/reports/statbriefs/sb205-Hospital-Discharge-Postacute-Care.pdf.

Wong, B. M., Etchells, E. E., Kuper, A., Levinson, W., & Shojania, K. G. (2010). Teaching quality improvement and patient safety to trainees: A systematic review. *Academic Medicine : Journal of the Association of American Medical Colleges*, *85*(9), 1425–1439. doi:10.1097/ACM.0b013e3181e2d0c6

Medical student reflections on geriatrics: Moral distress, empathy, ethics and end of life

Mary E. Camp ⓘ, Haekyung Jeon-Slaughter, Anne E. Johnson, and John Z. Sadler

ABSTRACT
Medical students' early clinical encounters may influence their perceptions of geriatrics. This study examines reflective essays written by 3rd-
year medical students on required clinical rotations. Using content
analysis, the authors analyzed the essays' thematic content. The authors
then used chi-squared analysis to compare themes with geriatric
patients (age 60+) to themes with other age groups. One hundred
twenty out of 802 essays described a geriatric patient. The most common geriatric themes were (1) death and dying, (2) decision making, (3)
meaningful physician–patient interactions, (4) quality of care, and (5)
professional development. Geriatric essays were more likely to discuss
death/dying and risk–benefit themes and less likely to discuss abuse.
Geriatric essays were more likely to describe students' moral distress.
Geriatric essays with moral distress were more likely to include empathy
themes compared to geriatric essays without moral distress. Geriatric
patients may pose unique ethical challenges for early clinical students.

Introduction

As the population of older adults continues to grow, the recruitment of medical students into geriatric specialties has become a prominent public health concern. An increasing body of literature examines the reasons that medical students either choose or avoid geriatric specialties (Meiboom, De Vries, Hertogh, & Scheele, 2015), with a focus on modifiable factors that could be addressed through education. For instance, trainees with more positive attitudes toward older adults are more likely to pursue geriatrics (Hughes et al., 2008; Schigelone, 2004), and positive experiences with older adults may shape these attitudes and interests (Briggs, Atkins, Playfer, & Corrado, 2006; Fitzgerald, Wray, Halter, Williams, & Supiano, 2003; Voogt, Mickus, Santiago, & Herman, 2008). Accordingly, many medical schools have implemented curriculum to encourage meaningful experiences with older adults (Gonzales, Morrow-Howell, & Gilbert, 2010; Laks et al., 2016; Lu, Hoffman, Hosokawa, Gray, & Zweig, 2010; Ray-Griffith, Krain, Messias, & Wilkins, 2016; Shue, McNeley, & Arnold, 2005). Others have published reports on geriatric-focused medical training that improves trainees' attitudes toward older patients or consideration of geriatric specialties (Goeldlin et al., 2014; Hughes et al., 2008).

Although this evidence makes a case for medical schools to bolster geriatric-specific clinical and educational programs, it does not account for the fact that medical students encounter older adults on general clinical services as part of their core clinical training.

Adults age 65 years or older have the highest health care utilization rates in the United States (National Center for Health Statistics, 2016), and students often encounter older adults as they rotate through general inpatient and outpatient services. Considering the relative paucity of geriatric specialists and the relative frequency of geriatric care visits, students are very likely to treat older adults with the supervision of someone who does not have specialized training in geriatric care.

Understanding these clinical encounters is critical to understanding how trainees experience the "real world" of geriatrics care during their formative years of clinical training. A growing trend in medical education uses qualitative analyses of students' reflective writing to better understand students' complex experiences (Chretien, Goldman, & Faselis, 2008; Cohn et al., 2009; Dyrbye, Harris, & Rohren, 2007; Karnieli-Miller et al., 2010; Kind, Everett, & Ottolini, 2009; Levine, Kern, & Wright, 2008; Lie, Shapiro, Cohn, & Najm, 2010; Mann, Gordon, & MacLeod, 2009; Martinez & Lo, 2008; Rosenbaum, Lobas, & Ferguson, 2005; Ross, Williams, Doran, & Lypson, 2010; Wear, 2002). Qualitative research in general has been recognized as a method by which researchers can take a deep and nuanced view of innovative questions related to geriatric care (Schoenberg & McAuley, 2007; Schoenberg, Miller, & Pruchno, 2011), and reflective writing exercises have been used to explore students' attitudes towards older adults in the context of geriatrics curriculum (Hsieh, Arenson, Eanes, & Sifri, 2010; Shield, Farrell, Campbell, Nanda, & Wetle, 2015; Westmoreland et al., 2009).

However, very little data describes medical students' actual encounters with older patients, especially during required clerkships in medical school (i.e., nongeriatric specialty settings). Two such studies examined students' experiences of geriatric patients on internal medicine clerkships. Higashi, Tillack, Steinman, Harper, and Johnston (2012) completed an ethnographic study of residents and medical students in two training hospitals over a 4-month period of time. The authors concluded that "most participants felt some combination of frustration and warmth toward older patients." In this study, trainees considered geriatrics as less rewarding in part because of "hidden curriculum" related to senior physicians' attitudes, negative views of aging, and other factors related to complex systems of care (Higashi et al., 2012). Another study of similar design by Meiboom, Diedrich et al. (2015) reported similar results. Medical students experienced geriatric patients as "frustrating and not interesting," and they observed negative attitudes by role models, particularly residents (Meiboom, Diedrich, Vries, Hertogh, & Scheele, 2015).

We were unable to find any study that examined interactions with older adults on other required services (such as surgery or neurology). We were also unable to find any study comparing early clinical experiences with geriatric patients to experiences with non-geriatric patients. This leaves a significant gap in the literature.

Therefore, in the context of a qualitative analysis of a large cohort of clerkship reflective essays, we were interested in exploring medical students' earliest and most formative clinical experiences with older adults. Specifically, we were interested in understanding how students encounter older adults across their entire scope of required clinical rotations and how these encounters may differ from those with younger patients.

This study asks the following research questions: (1) What ethical themes do students describe when interacting with geriatric patients? (2) Do these themes differ from those described with patients of other age groups? (3) Do students use the same level of self-reflection and ethical engagement when writing about geriatric patients and nongeriatric patients? (4) Do students describe the same level of moral distress when working with geriatric patients and nongeriatric patients?

These questions are key to understanding the medical trainee experience to allow more effective curriculum development and direct supervision of trainees during this important time in their medical education. These answers would also help educators address challenges that may prevent students from considering geriatric specialties.

Method

In 2009, the University of Texas Southwestern medical school clerkship curriculum rolled out a new initiative in which all 3rd-year clinical rotations (with the exception of psychiatry) required students to write a one-page reflective essay on an ethics or professionalism topic that the student encountered during the rotation. (The psychiatry clerkship had already instituted its own reflective essay rubric and for this reason was excluded from the school policy and this study.) After approval from the Institutional Review Board, we collected all essays that had been turned in to the course directors during the academic year. Students were notified of the study by e-mail and were given an opportunity to opt out if they chose to do so. An honest broker (individual not involved in data handling, analysis, and interpretation of data) deidentified the sample of essays to remove the name of the student author, identities of any patients, and the identities of any faculty or medical staff.

Quality indicators

Students were instructed to "write a one page reflection essay based on a clinical encounter or interpersonal encounter on the wards or clinics ... the goal is to capture a thought-provoking, affirming, or troubling experience during that clerkship." The students were also instructed to choose an experience with a related ethics theme.

In determining whether the students fulfilled these minimum assignment requirements, we analyzed them for two "quality indicators." First, we determined whether they described a personal experience from an introspective first-person point of view. We referred to these essays as having "I statements." These statements involve introspective statements such as "I thought," "I wondered," or "I felt." Simply telling a story using first-person pronouns (e.g., "I rotated at the pediatric hospital") would not be considered introspective.

In Mezirow's description of nonreflective versus reflective action, he defines *introspection* as "thinking about ourselves, our thoughts or feelings." In Mezirow's taxonomy, introspection is categorized as nonreflective because it does not involve validity testing of prior learning (Mezirow, 1991, p. 107–108). However, it is a prerequisite step for reflective action that may follow. We would hope that students would progress toward being better able to use critical reflection over time (i.e., not just thinking about oneself, but also using validity testing to transform thoughts or behaviors). However, we considered introspection as the minimum level at which we could ensure that they had engaged with the assignment.

Second, we determined whether or not the student had included an ethical theme. Those that excluded an ethical theme were classified as having "low ethical content." For instance, if a student merely presented a clinical scenario (such as an interesting diagnostic case) or stated his or her opinion (e.g., on dissatisfaction with a grade), these were placed in the "low ethical content" category.

Qualitative analysis of themes

We used content analysis to code the text and identify themes. Because existing research on this topic is extremely limited, we used inductive category development to establish our themes from the data directly. (Hsieh & Shannon, 2005). First, 24 randomly selected essays were read and used to develop our initial coding scheme. We then prospectively identified themes in an essay-by-essay case reading and review of the entire sample. Although some themes recurred in many essays, we continued to see new unique and relevant themes emerge as we continued with the analysis of all of the essays. Therefore, we continued to add new themes as they were identified. There was no limit to the number of distinct themes we identified in each essay. Some essays focused on only one theme, and others discussed many themes.

The scoring of the particular themes was done by consensus of two authors (JZS and MEC) in real time, and discrepancies were resolved as they arose during coding. A copy of the complete taxonomy of codes is available from the senior author (JZS). Following our initial coding, we then grouped our themes into broader thematic categories of related concepts.

We used NVivo 9.0 for storage and data management, but the analysis was done by reading and not by computer analysis. In this way, we were able to immerse ourselves in the material to obtain a richer analysis of the contents of the essays.

Moral distress

As noted above, we used an inductive coding approach for identification of themes. However, we had one exception. We were particularly interested in identifying "moral distress" in student essays, and we analyzed each essay for presence or absence of this theme.

Moral distress occurs when someone recognizes an ethically appropriate course of action but is unable to carry it out (Jameton, 1984). We coded essays as containing the moral distress theme when (1) a student described himself or herself doing or colluding with actions that the student believed were morally suspect or frankly immoral and (2) the student expressed that he or she was bothered by this to some degree.

Comparison of geriatric and nongeriatric essays

Because our research objectives include not only an exploration of experiences with older adults, but also a comparison with experiences with other age groups, we employed mixed methods to allow us to identify statistical differences between groups (Happ, 2009).

Using textual references, we separated essays describing older adults from those describing younger or age-unspecified patients. We refer to these as "geriatric essays" and "nongeriatric essays" respectively. The "geriatric essays" included those in which the student described an older adult or specified an age of 60 or older. Although age 65 years is sometimes used as the beginning of "geriatric" care, there is no absolute determinate in terms of chronological age. Globally, the World Health Organization and United Nations use age 60 years when describing older age (United Nations Department of Economic and Social Affairs, 2013; World Health Organization, 2015), as do other studies (Depp & Jeste, 2005; Stahl et al., 2017). We

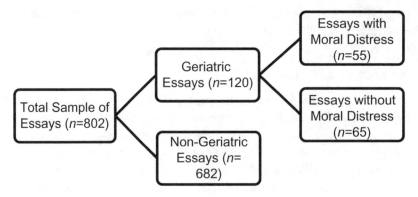

Figure 1. Grouping of essays for comparison of themes.

chose age 60 years because we felt that it was sufficient to ensure that the patient was of an older generation and to maximize our ability to capture information about interactions with this population.

We then compared the frequencies of themes in geriatric versus nongeriatric essays. All of the essays were included in this analysis, even those classified as "low ethical content."

For this purpose, when a theme appeared in an essay, we coded the essay as positive for that theme. The traditional chi-squared (χ^2) statistical test was used to determine which themes statistically associated with geriatric or nongeriatric essays. We limited our analysis to themes that occurred in 10% or more of the geriatric essays. One exception was the theme of "abuse" that appeared less often but was of particular relevance (as described in the Results section).

Within the sample of geriatric essays only, we then created two groups: essays with moral distress and essays without moral distress. We used the chi-squared test again to determine differences between themes in these two groups (Figure 1).

Results

Out of 802 total essays, 120 essays described an encounter with an older adult. The greatest number of geriatric essays came from individuals in internal medicine and the "unknown" clerkship categories, but geriatric essays were identified on every clerkship except for obstetrics/gynecology and pediatrics (Table 1).

Table 1. Number of geriatric essays per clerkship.

Clerkship	Number
Total	120
Internal medicine	45
Surgery	26
Family medicine	22
Neurology	12
Obstetrics and Gynecology	0
Pediatrics	0
Unspecified	15

Quality indicators

First, essays were evaluated for whether they used an introspective first person point of view, which we called the use of "I Statements." The vast majority of essays were written in this manner, including 87% of geriatric essays and 91.5% of nongeriatric essays. There was no statistically significant difference between these two groups. Second, if an essay was determined to lack ethical content, it was coded as "low ethical content." Only 5% of geriatric essays were coded as "low ethical content" versus. 12.5% nongeriatric essays, which represented a statistically significant difference (χ^2 49.9, $p < .001$).

Thematic content

Table 2 illustrates the themes most frequently discussed in the geriatric essays, which we have grouped into five thematic clusters:

(1) Death and dying: dying process, doing everything vs. letting die, DNR, and dying in the hospital. These themes all relate to a students' experience of a patient death. Each of these themes occurred more often in geriatric essays, compared to non-geriatric essays, and these differences reached statistical significance.

More than 25% of geriatric essays discussed the death of a patient, making "dying process" the most commonly described theme. Although students described their patients' death in a variety of ways, depending on the nature of the patient's illness or other psychosocial factors, these narratives predominantly described the death of a patient as a formative experience that would have a lasting impact on the student. In one example, a student stated:

Table 2. Commonly endorsed themes in geriatric versus nongeriatric essays.

	Frequency (% Geri Essays)	Frequency (% Nongeri Essays)	Chi-squared Value	p Value
Death and dying				
Dying process[a]	31 (25.8)	64 (9.4)	27.2	p < 0.001
Doing everything vs. letting die[a]	15 (12.5)	26 (3.8)	15.9	p < 0.001
Do Not Resuscitate[a]	12 (10.0)	22 (3.2)	11.5	0.001
Dying in the hospital[a]	12 (10.0)	26 (3.8)	8.7	0.003
Decision-making				
Risk–benefit analysis[a]	19 (15.8)	51 (7.5)	8.9	0.003
Disputes	13 (10.8)	57 (8.4)	0.8	0.38
Informed consent for care	13 (10.8)	100 (14.7)	1.2	0.27
Meaningful physician–patient interactions				
Empathy	19 (15.8)	122 (18.0)	0.3	0.59
Breaking bad news	13 (10.8)	50 (7.3)	1.7	0.19
Doctor–patient relationship	12 (10.0)	86 (12.6)	0.6	0.42
Quality of care				
Duty to comprehensive care	18 (15.0)	75 (11.0)	1.6	0.20
Adequate treatment	17 (14.2)	85 (12.5)	0.3	0.60
Physician responsibility	14 (11.7)	74 (10.9)	0.1	0.80
Allocation of resources	17 (14.2)	69 (10.1)	1.7	0.19
Professional development				
Role of medical student	18 (15.0)	95 (13.9)	0.1	0.76
Job well done	13 (10.8)	85 (12.5)	0.3	0.62

a. Statistical significance defined as $p < .05$.

No matter how hard I try, I will never be able to forget this gentleman: a man of 6 feet with a stature and appearance incongruent with someone who one would imagine would be bent over weeping over an elderly woman half his size. I will not forget that this elderly woman's mental status continued to deteriorate over the course of the night, and that she never made it. (dying process, dying in the hospital)

Another student describes his or her struggle to balance professional roles with personal feelings in the context of humanistic care:

My team was called to his room after he passed away, and as I slowly walked in to the room and heard the cries of Mr. T's children and gut wrenching sob of his wife, who was so frail and barely able to stand over her husband's dead body, I started crying I looked around to my resident and intern to see how exactly I should be responding at that moment as I had absolutely no idea what to do. I desperately wanted to console Mr. T's wife, who seemed like she was falling apart by the second, but I did not know whether the appropriate thing to do was pat her on her back, hug her, or say "I'm sorry." In the end, I decided not to do anything. I just stood quietly in the corner and took everything in. Some part of me felt that I needed to hold back my tears, but tears kept streaming down my face.

I looked around and noticed that while the other members of my team looked very saddened, I was the only one crying." (dying process, dying in the hospital)

Decision-Making: risk-benefit analysis, disputes, and informed consent for clinical care. This cluster encompasses student reflections on the process of clinical decision-making. Risk-benefit analysis refers to the weighing of risks and benefits of a clinical action

and this was the only theme in this cluster that reached a statistical association with geriatric essays. Disputes refers to a disagreement within the treatment team or between the treatment team and the patient or family. Informed consent for clinical care refers to the process of obtaining consent from a patient or surrogate family member.

In this thematic cluster, students often describe the challenges of providing care for patients with complex medical needs and surrogate decision makers. For example, one student reflected on the decision-making process that led a spouse to consent to a surgery for a patient who did not survive postoperatively:

Mr. S. was found unresponsive later that night by the nurse. A full code was run and the initial rhythm strip showed no electrical activity and was later pronounced dead, presumably from arrhythmia or other post-op complications (MI/CVA/PE). His wife would later arrive at the hospital. I cannot imagine how she could have felt. It was a very difficult decision for her to agree with the surgery and she post-operatively she felt she had made the best decision, even against her husband's wants. (risk–benefit analysis)

(3) Meaningful physician–patient interactions: empathy, breaking bad news, and,doctor–patient relationship. This cluster refers to situations where the student experienced an influential or memorable interpersonal interaction with the patient. Empathy themes occurred when the student explicitly expressed that he or she felt what the patient was feeling or experienced what they thought it would be like to be in that patient's situation. Breaking bad news refers to the formative experience of sharing a poor prognosis or other difficult material with a patient or family. Doctor–patient relationship themes were coded when the student specifically commented on this important relationship in a personal way.

In this thematic cluster, students often described getting to know their patients as real people who experienced conditions that the student had previously only known through textbooks. One student describes his or her awakening to the realities of some patients living with Parkinson's disease:

Parkinson's disease is a horrible disease, but I did not realize just how devastating it could be. The disease progression affects everyone differently, and unfortunately my patient, Mr. A, was one of those who had a more severe form. I tried to put myself in his shoes, and believe me, it felt uncomfortable. I tried to imagine myself the way I am: semi-intelligent, conscious and aware of my surroundings, but instead of being able to move around, I am trapped in a body that has been switched "off," unable to move, see, or talk, all the while the rest of the world is going on without me. (empathy)

(4) Quality of care: duty to comprehensive care, adequate treatment, physician responsibility, and allocation of resources. This cluster includes students' descriptions of how well the student, other practitioners, or the larger system cared for patients' complex medical or psychosocial needs.

Although the students typically held a high view of the responsibility of the physician, they also encountered systems issues, financial hardships, and other challenges that limited their ability to provide the level of care they aspired to:

The most touching example was that of Mr. J, a 64-year-old Parkinson's patient who had been on hospice care previously. However, he had been denied renewal after 6 months because he was no longer considered a suitable candidate. The wife of the patient informed me that it was because "he is not dying soon enough. (allocation of resources)

(5) Professional development: role of medical student and job well done. This cluster refers to student descriptions of their own role in the medical team or on the observation of role models.

Although the students were often frustrated with their perceived lack of autonomy or position in the hierarchical system of medical education, they also identified others on the treatment team that provided an example that the student praised or desired to emulate:

Professionally, I believe my team did an excellent job. Speaking with the family in an honest and straightforward fashion I believe is the best approach in disclosing a diagnosis. The level of care was excellent, multiple specialists were consulted and the treatment being implemented was the cumulative input of many physicians. (job well done)

Abuse

The theme of abuse was not included in the most common themes, as it was described in only 1.7% of geriatric essays, compared to 7.8% of nongeriatric essays. Abuse (which includes neglect) was the only theme that was statistically associated with nongeriatric essays. Out of 55 total mentions of patient abuse, the majority described abuse of a child ($n = 36$), followed by abuse of a woman ($n = 17$). A minority described elder abuse ($n = 2$). Child Protective Services reporting was mentioned 22 times, and Adult Protective Services reporting was not mentioned once.

Moral distress and empathy

Forty-six percent of geriatric essays described moral distress, compared to 32% of non-geriatric essays. This represents a significant difference (χ^2 8.542, $p = .003$).

The moral distress essays involved many of the themes reported above. For example, one student reflected on the death of a patient and medical decision making:

> At one in the afternoon, when the day was getting really busy the bad news came in that Mr. K had died in the OR. This came as shock to me. I did not know what to make of it. I felt bad because if I had not pushed surgery to do the surgery sooner he would still be alive at least for the next two days. I was also angry at surgery, because they did not act sooner and this was a surgical emergency. For the rest of that call day I thought about these issues.

This student describes moral distress in the form of "anger" at constraints placed by other services. However, the student also expresses uncertainty about whether his or her own actions were actually in the best interest of the patient. Other students vividly described moral distress at being unable to take action in an area where the student felt moral certainty:

> As I stood there listening to the younger daughter recount her illness and parallel it to her mother, I was screaming inside, "No! Your mother is 80-something, and even though you went through a rough time, this is not the same. Your mother will die sometime, and the question on the table now is more like how long are we going to draw out her death." But I stood there with the most neutral expression on my face that I could have.

Within the geriatric essays, we separated those with moral distress ($n = 55$) from those without ($n = 65$). We then compared themes between the two groups. The only significant difference was empathy, which was more common in geriatric essays describing moral distress and less common in essays without moral distress ($\chi^2 = 7.1$, $p = .0079$). No other themes reached a statistical significance.

Discussion and implications

Our literature review indicated that this is the first study of medical students' reflective essays comparing thematic content in essays involving geriatric patients with essays involving all other age groups. As such, it offers a unique window into clerkship students' thinking about geriatrics and raises some ideas about geriatric education for medical students.

In our sample, students describe older adults with ethical and moral sensitivity. In fact, students were actually more ethically descriptive when discussing geriatric encounters (as evidenced by lower occurrences of "low ethical content"). These are interesting findings in light of prior reports of students describing geriatrics as "boring" or "not interesting" (Higashi et al., 2012; Meiboom, Diedrich et al., 2015). In our sample, students had a lot to say about the complex scenarios that occurred in the context of geriatric care.

Further, students described more moral distress when discussing encounters with geriatric patients, compared to encounters with younger patients. This finding is striking because it indicates that not only did students recognize ethical challenges associated with geriatrics care, but also that they were personally affected by these challenges.

Of particular interest, within the group of geriatric essays, the essays describing moral distress also described higher levels of empathy. We wonder whether this represents a reporting phenomenon or an experience phenomenon. Reporting reflects that students who are able to articulate moral distress are also better able to articulate empathy. Alternatively, it is possible that students who are more attuned to their own empathic feelings are actually more likely to experience moral distress. In this case, students who experience empathic reactions to older adults in particular may also be subject to higher levels of moral distress while working with these older adults. It would seem that the ability to empathically "connect" with older adults would attract a student to geriatric specialties, but we do not know whether the associated moral distress might serve as a deterrent. In either case, we do know from the literature that moral distress is associated with burnout, turnover, and poorer professional quality of life (Austin, Saylor, & Finley, 2016; Piers et al., 2012). This may indicate that educators should address the potential for moral distress in concert with discussing empathic reactions to geriatric patients. Students who are more naturally empathic may need additional support or training in how to manage and address moral distress in themselves and others.

In comparing themes in geriatric essays to other essays, themes pertaining to death and dying were statistically associated with geriatric essays. This should not be surprising because older adults have significantly higher death rates than other age groups (National Center for Health Statistics, 2010), and approximately 75% of hospital deaths occur in individuals age 65 years or older (National Center for Health Statistics, 2013). This is also consistent with previous reports that students may equate geriatrics care with end-of-life care, which may make the field less appealing for those who would rather focus on "cure" than "care" (Higashi et al., 2012). In our study, the parallel finding of prominent death and dying themes along with high moral distress suggests that our students may not be fully ready to recognize and deal with the humanistic and ethical challenges of end-of-life care in the geriatric population. Considering that these essays represent students' earliest exposures to patients, the preponderance of death and dying themes and moral distress themes raise questions about our students' experiences with geriatric patients being overly negative. Given the literature that encourages positive early experiences with older adults, our findings of students having negative experiences is worrisome for future recruitment of students into geriatrics careers.

Risk–benefit themes were also statistically associated with geriatric essays. Risk–benefit themes were dominated by concerns about risks and benefits of treatment options. To our surprise, end-of-life care themes regarding risk benefit were relatively uncommon. However, this finding does reflect the complexity of geriatric patients, for whom complicated medical comorbidities, impaired decision-making capacity, and other social factors may make medical decisions less straightforward. In our students' reporting, these complicated risk–benefit questions were reported more often with older adults than younger patients.

The last theme that was significantly different between geriatric and nongeriatric essays was abuse (which also included neglect). This was the only theme that was significantly more common in nongeriatric essays, indicating that students were not recognizing or not discussing elder abuse. The discrepancy between discussions of child and elder abuse is particularly striking because we know that both are common occurrences in potentially vulnerable populations. According to the Texas Department of Family and Protective Services (DFPS; 2015), the incidence of abuse is 8.9 per 1000 for adult cases, and 9.1 per 1000 for children. We know from the literature that practitioners and students often do not detect elder abuse (Fisher, Rudd, Walker, & Stewart, 2016; Thompson-McCormick, Jones, Cooper, & Livingston, 2009), and by one meta-analysis, as many as one half of detected cases go unreported (Cooper, Selwood, & Livingston, 2009). Our findings are consistent with others reported in the literature, in that our sample of students either did not recognize elder abuse, or they recognized it and chose not to write about it.

This study has several limitations. Although we collected a large number of reflective essays, our sample is only from a single academic medical center, limiting the generalizability of our findings. The absolute numbers of geriatric essays was relatively small compared to the entire sample, making for weak statistical power in looking at comparisons with other moderate and low frequency themes. The bulk of our students' essays responded to our instructions for professionally or ethically significant themes by describing ethical or professional problems. It is possible that a motivation toward negative moral themes may impose an artificially negative halo effect on the interpretation of our data. Lastly, in this sample we were unable to include ethnographic correlations because of stipulations of anonymity for the student authors. Future research could explore these additional factors.

This study presents many avenues for continued research. First, the finding of prominent moral distress themes indicates a need for additional study on moral distress and specialty choice or career satisfaction in geriatrics specifically. Second, our findings reveal potential needs of students working with older patients. Additional research on educational interventions in the core clerkships would help educators better know how to address these challenges with students in an evidence-based manner.

Acknowledgments

The authors would like to acknowledge Dr. James Wagner, Dr. Celia Jenkins, and Heather Smith for their contributions to the educational programs described in this article.

Disclosure statement

No potential conflict of interest was reported by the authors.

ORCID

Mary E. Camp http://orcid.org/0000-0001-7997-0058

References

Austin, C. L., Saylor, R., & Finley, P. J. (2016). Moral distress in physicians and nurses: Impact on professional quality of life and turnover. *Psychol Trauma: Theory, Research, Practice, and Policy, 9* (4), 399–406. doi:10.1037/tra0000201

Briggs, S., Atkins, R., Playfer, J., & Corrado, O. J. (2006). Why do doctors choose a career in geriatric medicine? *Clinical Medica (Lond), 6*(5), 469–472. doi:10.7861/clinmedicine.6-5-469

Chretien, K., Goldman, E., & Faselis, C. (2008). The reflective writing class blog: Using technology to promote reflection and professional development. *Journal of General Internal Medicine, 23* (12), 2066–2070. doi:10.1007/s11606-008-0796-5

Cohn, F. G., Shapiro, J., Lie, D. A., Boker, J., Stephens, F., & Leung, L. A. (2009). Interpreting values conflicts experienced by obstetrics-gynecology clerkship students using reflective writing. *Academic Medicine, 84*(5), 587–596. doi:10.1097/ACM.0b013e31819f6ecc

Cooper, C., Selwood, A., & Livingston, G. (2009). Knowledge, detection, and reporting of abuse by health and social care professionals: A systematic review. *American Journal of Geriatric Psychiatry, 17*(10), 826–838. doi:10.1097/JGP.0b013e3181b0fa2e

Depp, C., & Jeste, D. (2005). Definitions and predictors of successful aging: A comprehensive review of larger quantitative studies. *American Journal of Geriatric Psychiatry, 14*(1), 6–20. doi:10.1097/01.JGP.0000192501.03069.bc

Dyrbye, L. N., Harris, I., & Rohren, C. H. (2007). Early clinical experiences from students' perspectives: A qualitative study of narratives. *Academic Medicine, 82*(10), 979–988. doi:10.1097/ACM.0b013e318149e29c

Fisher, J. M., Rudd, M. P., Walker, R. W., & Stewart, J. (2016). Training tomorrow's doctors to safeguard the patients of today: using medical student simulation training to explore barriers to recognition of elder abuse. *Journal of the American Geriatrics Society, 64*(1), 168–173. doi:10.1111/jgs.13875

Fitzgerald, J. T., Wray, L. A., Halter, J. B., Williams, B. C., & Supiano, M. A. (2003). Relating medical students' knowledge, attitudes, and experience to an interest in geriatric medicine. *Gerontologist, 43*(6), 849–855. doi:10.1093/geront/43.6.849

Goeldlin, A. O., Siegenthaler, A., Moser, A., Stoeckli, Y. D., Stuck, A. E., & Schoenenberger, A. W. (2014). Effects of geriatric clinical skills training on the attitudes of medical students. *BMC Medical Education, 14*, 233. doi:10.1186/1472-6920-14-233

Gonzales, E., Morrow-Howell, N., & Gilbert, P. (2010). Changing medical students' attitudes toward older adults. *Gerontology & Geriatrics Education, 31*(3), 220–234. doi:10.1080/02701960.2010.503128

Happ, M. B. (2009). Mixed methods in gerontological research. *Research in Gerontological Nursing, 2*(2), 122–127. doi:10.3928/19404921-20090401-06

Hall M. J., Levant, S., & DeFrances, C. J (2013). *Trends in inpatient hospital deaths: National hospital discharge survey, 2000-2010*(NCHS data brief, no 118). Hyattsville, MD, USA: National Center for Health Statistics. Retrieved from http://www.cdc.gov/nchs/data/databriefs/db118.htm

Higashi, R. T., Tillack, A. A., Steinman, M., Harper, M., & Johnston, C. B. (2012). Elder care as "frustrating" and "boring": Understanding the persistence of negative attitudes toward older patients among physicians-in-training. *Journal of Aging Studies, 26*(4), 476–483. doi:10.1016/j.jaging.2012.06.007

Hsieh, C., Arenson, C. A., Eanes, K., & Sifri, R. D. (2010). Reflections of medical students regarding the care of geriatric patients in the continuing care retirement community. *Journal of the American Medical Directors Association, 11*(7), 506–510. doi:10.1016/j.jamda.2009.11.001

Hsieh, H., & Shannon, S. E. (2005). The approaches to qualitative content analysis. *Qualitative Health Research, 15*(9), 1277–1288. doi:10.1177/1049732305276687

Hughes, N. J., Soiza, R. L., Chua, M., Hoyle, G. E., MacDonald, A., Primrose, W. R., & Seymour, D. G. (2008). Medical student attitudes toward older people and willingness to consider a career in geriatric medicine. *Journal of the American Geriatrics Society, 56*(2), 334–338. doi:10.1111/j.1532-5415.2007.01552.x

Jameton, A. (1984). *Nursing practice: The ethical issues.* Englewood Cliffs, NJ: Prentice Hall.

Karnieli-Miller, O., Taylor, A. C., Cottingham, A. H., Inui, T. S., Vu, T. R., & Frankel, R. M. (2010). Exploring the meaning of respect in medical student education: An analysis of student narratives. *Journal of General Internal Medicine, 25*(12), 1309–1314. doi:10.1007/s11606-010-1471-1

Kind, T., Everett, V. R., & Ottolini, M. (2009). Learning to connect: Students' reflections on doctor-patient interactions. *Patient Education and Counseling, 75*(2), 149–154. doi:10.1016/j.pec.2008.09.011

Laks, J., Wilson, L. A., Khandelwal, C., Footman, E., Jamison, M., & Roberts, E. (2016). Service-Learning in Communities of Elders (SLICE): Development and evaluation of an introductory geriatrics course for medical students. *Teaching and Learning in Medicine, 28*(2), 210–218. doi:10.1080/10401334.2016.1146602

Levine, R. B., Kern, D. E., & Wright, S. M. (2008). The impact of prompted narrative writing during internship on reflective practice: A qualitative study. *Advances in Health Sciences Education : Theory and Practice, 13*(5), 723–733. doi:10.1007/s10459-007-9079-x

Lie, D., Shapiro, J., Cohn, F., & Najm, W. (2010). Reflective practice enriches clerkship students' cross-cultural experiences. *Journal of General Internal Medicine*, *25*(Suppl 2), S119–125. doi:10.1007/s11606-009-1205-4

Lu, W., Hoffman, K., Hosokawa, M., Gray, P., & Zweig, S. (2010). First year medical students' knowledge, attitudes, and interest in geriatric medicine. *Educational Gerontology*, *36*(8), 687–701. doi:10.1080/03601270903534630

Mann, K., Gordon, J., & MacLeod, A. (2009). Reflection and reflective practice in health professions education: A systematic review. *Advances in Health Sciences Education : Theory and Practice*, *14* (4), 595–621. doi:10.1007/s10459-007-9090-2

Martinez, W., & Lo, B. (2008). Medical students' experiences with medical errors: An analysis of medical student essays. *Medical Education*, *42*(7), 733–741. doi:10.1111/j.1365-2923.2008.03109.x

Meiboom, A., Diedrich, C., Vries, H. D., Hertogh, C., & Scheele, F. (2015). The hidden curriculum of the medical care for elderly patients in medical education: A qualitative study. *Gerontology & Geriatrics Education*, *36*(1), 30–44. doi:10.1080/02701960.2014.966902

Meiboom, A. A., De Vries, H., Hertogh, C. M., & Scheele, F. (2015). Why medical students do not choose a career in geriatrics: A systematic review. *BMC Medical Education*, *15*, 101. doi:10.1186/s12909-015-0384-4

Mezirow, J. (1991). *Transformative dimensions of adult learning* (1st ed.). San Francisco, CA, USA: Jossey-Bass.

National Center for Health Statistics. (2010). *Worktable 23R. Death rates by 10-year age groups: United States and each state, 2007*. Atlanta, GA, USA: Centers for DiseaseControl and Prevention/National Center for Health Statistics Retrieved from http://www.cdc.gov/nchs/data/dvs/mortfinal2007_worktable23r.pdf

National Center for Health Statistics. (2016). *Health, United States, 2015: With special features on racial and ethnic health disparities. Hyattsville, MD: Author*. Retrieved from https://www.cdc.gov/nchs/data/hus/hus15.pdf#081

Piers, R. D., Van Den Eynde, M., Steeman, E., Vlerick, P., Benoit, D. D., & Van Den Noortgate, N. J. (2012). End-of-life care of the geriatric patient and nurses' moral distress. *Journal of the American Medical Directors Association*, *13*(1), 80, e87–13. doi:10.1016/j.jamda.2010.12.014

Ray-Griffith, S. L., Krain, L., Messias, E., & Wilkins, K. M. (2016). Fostering medical student interest in geriatrics and geriatric psychiatry. *Academic Psychiatry*, *40*(6), 960–961. doi:10.1007/s40596-015-0431-9

Rosenbaum, M. E., Lobas, J., & Ferguson, K. (2005). Using reflection activities to enhance teaching about end-of-life care. *Journal of Palliative Medicine*, *8*(6), 1186–1195. doi:10.1089/jpm.2005.8.1186

Ross, P. T., Williams, B. C., Doran, K. M., & Lypson, M. L. (2010). First-year medical students' perceptions of physicians' responsibilities toward the underserved: An analysis of reflective essays. *Journal of the National Medical Association*, *102*(9), 761–765. doi:10.1016/S0027-9684(15)30672-6

Schigelone, A. (2004). Some of my best friends are old: A qualitative exploration of medical students' interest in geriatrics. *Educational Gerontology*, *30*(8), 643–661. doi:10.1080/03601270490483887

Schoenberg, N. E., & McAuley, W. (2007). Promoting qualitative research. *The Gerontologist*, *51*, 576–577. doi:10.1093/geront/47.5.576

Shield, R. R., Farrell, T. W., Campbell, S. E., Nanda, A., & Wetle, T. (2015). Professional development and exposure to geriatrics: Medical student perspectives from narrative journals. *Gerontology & Geriatrics Education*, *36*(2), 144–160. doi:10.1080/02701960.2014.954043

Shue, C. K., McNeley, K., & Arnold, L. (2005). Changing medical students' attitudes about older adults and future older patients. *Academic Medicine*, *80*(10 Suppl), S6–9. doi:10.1097/00001888-200510001-00005

Stahl, S. T., Albert, S. M., Dew, M. A., Anderson, S., Karp, J. F., Gildengers, A. G., … Reynolds, C. F. (2017). Measuring participant effort in a depression prevention trial: Who engages in problem-solving therapy? *American Journal of Geriatric Psychiatry*, *25*(8), 909–916. doi:10.1016/j.jagp.2017.03.005

Texas Department of Family and Protective Services. (2015). *Annual report and data book*. Retrieved from https://www.dfps.state.tx.us/About_DFPS/Annual_Report/2015/pdf/DFPS_2015_Annual_Report_and_Databook.pdf

Thompson-McCormick, J., Jones, L., Cooper, C., & Livingston, G. (2009). Medical students' recognition of elder abuse. *International Journal of Geriatric Psychiatry*, *24*(7), 770–777. doi:10.1002/gps.2209

United Nations Department of Economic and Social Affairs. (2013). *World population ageing*. Retrieved from http://www.un.org/en/development/desa/population/publications/pdf/ageing/WorldPopulationAgeing2013.pdf

Voogt, S. J., Mickus, M., Santiago, O., & Herman, S. E. (2008). Attitudes, experiences, and interest in geriatrics of first-year allopathic and osteopathic medical students. *Journal of the American Geriatrics Society*, *56*(2), 339–344. doi:10.1111/j.1532-5415.2007.01541.x

Wear, D. (2002). "Face-to-face with It": Medical students' narratives about their end-of-life education. *Academic Medicine*, *77*(4), 271–277. doi:10.1097/00001888-200204000-00003

Westmoreland, G. R., Counsell, S. R., Sennour, Y., Schubert, C. C., Frank, K. I., Wu, J., . . . Inui, T. S. (2009). Improving medical student attitudes toward older patients through a "council of elders" and reflective writing experience. *Journal of the American Geriatrics Society*, *57*(2), 315–320. doi:10.1111/j.1532-5415.2008.02102.x

World Health Organization. (2015). *World report on ageing and health*. Retrieved from http://apps.who.int/iris/bitstream/10665/186463/1/9789240694811_eng.pdf?ua=1

Schoenberg, N. E., Miller, E. A., & Pruchno, R. (2011). The qualitative portfolio at The Gerontologist: Strong and getting stronger. *Gerontologist*, *51*(3), 281–284. doi:10.1093/geront/gnr032

Addressing sexual health in geriatrics education

Mark Brennan-Ing, Liz Seidel, Pam Ansell, Barrie L. Raik, Debra Greenberg, Catherine Nicastri, Jennifer Breznay, Stephen E. Karpiak and Ronald D. Adelman

ABSTRACT

Adults remain sexually active well into later life, but few report discussing sexual health with a physician after age 50. The authors explored how geriatrics education might better address sexual health in the context of a psychosocial conference for geriatrics fellows, program directors, and faculty comprising an informational plenary, which included a skills-building presentation on taking sexual histories, and a program director/faculty roundtable. Although informed about older adult sexual health, knowledge scores of geriatrics fellows increased following the plenary. Fellows reported inconsistent sexual history taking with older adults and noted patient differences in age and gender as barriers. The roundtable discussion highlighted several barriers to inclusion of sexual health content in geriatrics curricula including competing competencies, lack of educational materials, and discomfort with this topic on the part of faculty. Implications of these findings for geriatrics training and education programs and suggestions for improving this domain of geriatrics education are discussed.

Introduction

Sexuality is an integral component of human life, affecting not only physical, but mental, social, and cultural interactions for people of all ages (Dominguez & Barbagallo, 2016). Although modes of sexual expression may change across the life course, sexual needs of older adults are like those of younger people per Dominguez and Barbagallo (2016). These authors elucidate several myths around sexuality and aging, including that sex does not exist in old age, sex among older adults is comical and disgusting, and that same-sex sexual behavior does not occur among older adults. Some of these myths are deeply rooted in social and cultural attitudes. Yet research finds that humans remain sexually active in old age. As people age, sexual activity may change from the emphasis on insertive intercourse to include nonpenetrative modes of sexual expression such as sexual touching and other forms of intimacy (Dominguez & Barbagallo, 2016).

In a national probability sample of adults between ages 57 and 85 years, Lindau et al. (2007) defined *sexual activity* as "any mutually voluntary activity with another person that involves sexual contact, whether or not intercourse or orgasm occurs." This study found that though there were declines with age, 73% of 57- to 64-year-olds were sexually active, as compared with 53% of 65- to 74-year-olds, and 26% of those between ages 75 and 85. Data from the 2012 General Social Survey finds 92% of adults 55 and older being sexually active in the past year (Amin, 2016). These findings reiterate earlier reports from the National Survey of Families and Households, that found that 53% of adults older than age 60 were sexually active in the past month (Marsiglio & Donnelly, 1991). Despite being sexually active, there is evidence that the sexual health of older adults is not being addressed in clinical settings. In the Lindau study, only 38% of men and 22% of women said they had talked to a physician about sex after age 50 (Lindau et al., 2007). In contrast, an observational study of 253 adolescents and their physicians found that sexual issues were discussed at 65% of office visits (Alexander et al., 2014).

This article describes an effort to better understand the role geriatrics education may play in addressing older adult sexual health. There is more than sufficient justification for health care providers to address the sexual health of their patients in clinical settings. Due to age-related physiological changes, many older adults experience sexual problems such as erectile dysfunction or low libido, which are sometimes related to other comorbidities (Minkin, 2016). Further, by continuing to be sexually active, older adults are at risk for sexually transmitted infections (STIs), such as the human immunodeficiency virus (HIV), syphilis, gonorrhea, and chlamydia.

Sexuality, health, and aging

There is a strong relationship between sexual activity in older adults and self-rated health (Hughes, Rostant, & Pelon, 2015; Lindau et al., 2007); those rating their health as "excellent" or "very good" are significantly more likely to be sexually active compared to those with "fair" or "poor" health. This finding reflects the connection between general health and sexual problems in later life. In a study of women age 60 and older, poor self-rated health was significantly related to sexual problems such as lack of interest or loss of sexual pleasure (Hughes et al., 2015). Regarding specific conditions, older women with diabetes are less likely to report being sexually active (Lindau et al., 2007), and being a survivor of gynecological or breast cancer may increase the risk of certain sexual problems like vulvovaginal atrophy and lack of sexual interest (Minkin, 2016). Among older men, prostate cancer is related to a variety of sexual problems including erectile dysfunction, urinary incontinence, and bowel incontinence (Minkin, 2016). Diabetes is also significantly related to the likelihood of erectile dysfunction (Lindau et al., 2007). Levels of sexual activity may also portend later health problems. Cross-lagged longitudinal analysis finds that high sexual frequency is associated with increased likelihood of future cardiovascular events in men, but in women, is associated with decreased risk of cardiovascular disease (Liu, Waite, Shen, & Wang, 2016). Other research suggests that sexually active older adults have better functional status and mood compared to their sexually inactive peers (Dominguez & Barbagallo, 2016).

Sexual problems in older women

Older women are less likely to report being sexually active compared to older men, which is related to the lack of sexual partner availability due to the growing gender imbalance and lower life expectancy of men in late life. Lindau et al. (2007) noted this pattern across all older age groups. This gender difference decreased sharply when comparing only married/partnered men and women. Older women in Lindau et al.'s (2007) study were also more likely to report they considered sex to be unimportant compared to men. Perceiving sex as not being important was also more common among those who were not sexually active.

Beyond psychosocial issues, there are a number of physiological changes that older women experience due to menopause and concomitant changes in hormone levels. Vaginal dryness or lack of lubrication is the most commonly reported physical sexual problem among older women, followed by inability to climax, finding sex not to be pleasurable, and pain during intercourse (Dominguez & Barbagallo, 2016; Hughes et al., 2015; Lindau et al., 2007). Lindau et al. (2007) found an inverse relationship among older women between better self-rated health and reports of experiencing sexual problems.

Sexual problems in older men
Among older men, erectile dysfunction is the most commonly reported problem, followed by lack of interest in sex, climaxing too quickly, anxiety about sexual performance, and the inability to climax (Dominguez & Barbagallo, 2016; Lindau et al., 2007). In addition to the impact of other health conditions, erectile dysfunction is related to levels of physical activity and leanness (Dominguez & Barbagallo, 2016).

Sexual problem overview
Lindau et al. (2007) report that approximately one half of the men and women in their sample reported at least one bothersome sexual problem and one third reported at least two such problems. Relatively small proportions of men (14%) and women (1%) said they were taking prescription or nonprescription medications/supplements to improve sexual function in the past year. In addition, participants in Lindau et al.'s (2007) study demonstrated a stronger association between physical health and sexual problems compared to the impact of age alone. Approximately one fourth of sexually active older adults in this study with a sexual problem avoided sex. Hughes et al. (2015) replicated earlier findings that sexual problems in older women were correlated with lower levels of life satisfaction and greater depressive symptoms.

Risks for STIs among older adults

Sexual dysfunction is not the sole health issue that confronts sexually active older adults. By continuing to engage in sexual activity, older adults are also at risk for acquiring STIs. This risk may be heightened by physiological changes associated with aging. Age-related weakening of the immune system (i.e., immunosenescence) makes it more difficult for older adults to fight infections (Pera et al., 2015), including STIs. For older men, erectile dysfunction may render the effective and consistent use of male condoms problematic. For older women who are postmenopausal, thinning of the vaginal walls and increased likelihood of tearing during sex make them particularly susceptible to STIs, especially HIV. Additionally, older women may not think of using condoms after menopause when pregnancy is no longer a concern (Patel, Gillespie, & Foxman, 2003). Rates of condom use with regular and casual partners decline with age (Reece et al., 2010) and are low for older adults regardless of gender (e.g., 13%–24%; Amin, 2016; Schick et al., 2010).

Similar to younger adults, older adults engage in behaviors that increase their risk for STIs, including having casual sex and multiple sexual partners, injecting drugs, using alcohol and drugs during sex, having male-to-male sex, and engaging sex workers (Amin, 2016; Golub et al., 2010; Milrod & Monto, 2016). Using Medicare claims data, Smith and Christakis (2009) found that widowhood increased the risk of STI diagnoses among men, but not among women. Further, these authors found that the risk of STIs among widowed men increased after the introduction of erectile dysfunction medications in the late 1990s by enabling men to remain sexually active. Further, older men continue to employ sex workers. Milrod and Monto (2016) studied older men between ages 60 and 84 who were clients of sex workers. Although recent insertive penile-vaginal sex without a male or female condom was reported by a small minority (3%), about one half of these men said they had engaged in this activity with a sex worker at least once. A history of condomless sex with a sex worker was related to preferences for sexual providers who did not require condoms, a previous diagnosis of an STI, and high perceived HIV risk. Less than one half of participants in this study reported using a male or female condom for all sexual acts, including oral sex.

Sexuality, older adults, and geriatricians

Given that older adults remain sexually active and face challenges to their sexual health due to aging and engaging in risky behaviors, it is imperative that sexual health be better addressed by health providers who serve older adults including geriatricians. How aware are geriatricians of important issues concerning sexuality in later life? How often do geriatricians take sexual histories and discuss sexual health with their older patients? How can existing geriatrics educational resources be leveraged to better address the sexual health needs of older adults? Answers to these questions were explored in a psychosocial educational forum for geriatric fellows.

The New York Metropolitan Area Geriatrics Consortium conference

As illustrated in the literature review, sexual health issues for older adults span physical, psychological, and social domains. Geriatricians should be competent in exploring and treating their patient's sexual concerns and problems, but may not be adequately trained or comfortable engaging these topics. In order to improve training of geriatric fellows in sexual health, the New York Metropolitan Area Consortium to Strengthen Psychosocial Education in Geriatric Fellowships held its annual conference highlighting sexual health in older adults.

The Consortium is an initiative to bring together geriatrics fellowship programs in the New York metropolitan area to develop and share psychosocial education. The Consortium highlights psychosocial issues affecting care of older adults, shares interinstitutional resources, and energizes geriatrics fellowship program directors and faculty to collaborate on creative and practical psychosocial curricula development. Each year approximately 50 geriatric fellows and 30 medical faculty and health professionals representing 20 academic medical institutions from New York, New Jersey, Connecticut, and Pennsylvania gather in Manhattan for a half-day conference that highlights a selected psychosocial topic area. Past topics have included grief, spirituality, elder abuse, and health literacy. The program includes a plenary session followed by case-based workshops coled by faculty from different disciplines and has been well received by fellows and faculty. In addition, the program directors and other faculty participate in a roundtable discussion and work throughout the year to collaboratively develop successful strategies, curriculum, and tools to enhance psychosocial educational modules. Details of this educational forum have been reported elsewhere (Adelman et al., 2011).

The Consortium Project Planning Committee, comprising members from five fellowship programs, considers psychosocial topic ideas for the annual conference that are chosen by consensus. The Project Planning Committee recognized that sexual health was an area in which trainees needed more education and communication skill-building strategies. Faculty also concluded it was an area that could be improved in their own practice. The conference plenary session provided fellows with evidence-based information on the importance of sexuality in aging and reviewed techniques for taking a sexual history. The geriatric fellows completed pre- and posttests on knowledge and attitudes about older adult sexuality and provided information about their current practices regarding taking sexual histories with older patients during the plenary session.

A roundtable forum for program directors, faculty, and other health professionals used the plenary session as the basis for developing a curriculum on understanding sexuality and sexual history taking, and participants were offered the opportunity of continuing to work on the project after the conference. A focus group of the program directors, faculty, and other health professionals was conducted prior to the roundtable forum to explore opportunities and barriers for incorporating sexual health content in geriatrics education. This article discusses the responses of the fellows to the "Sexuality and the Older Adult" plenary session, as well as information from the roundtable session focus group with program directors, faculty and other health professionals.

Method

Participants

Nineteen of the 20 Consortium programs were represented at the eighth annual psychosocial conference that focused on sexual health. Of the 85 attendees, 54 were geriatrics fellows, eight were Consortium faculty who facilitated four case-based psychosocial workshops for fellows, and 28 were program directors, faculty, and other health care professionals who attended the roundtable session.

Procedures

Plenary session

Data collection procedures, forms and protocols were approved by the Gay Men's Health Crisis (GMHC) Institutional Review Board. Geriatric fellows received an information packet upon their arrival at the conference that contained the informed consent document and the pre- and posttest. Originally, we planned to collect the pre- and posttest data using an audience response system, which would have automatically captured and tracked individual fellows' responses. Due to last-minute bad weather that interfered with staff travel, we were unable to use the audience response system and resorted to hard copies instead. Given the time constraints, we were unable to assign participant ID numbers to the hardcopies, and thus were unable to analyze pre- to posttest change using repeated measures statistics (i.e., paired t test). In addition, the poor weather was also responsible for several fellows arriving late for the symposium, and they were unable to provide pretest data (pretest $N = 28$; posttest $N = 34$). At the start of the conference, a description of the agenda was provided including the reasons for the data collection and the use of these data. Fellows then provided written informed consent and completed the pretest. Following the conference presentation, the posttest was completed.

Roundtable discussion forum focus group

A focus group of geriatric program directors (n = 14), faculty (n = 7), and other health professionals (n = 6) was held to gain more detailed insight into addressing sexual health issues in older adults. Prior to participation, focus group participants provided written informed consent, including permission for audio recording. A brief introduction was provided regarding the purpose of the focus group and how the data would be used. All roundtable discussion forum attendees participated. One of the authors who facilitated the focus group posed the following three questions:

(1) Does your fellowship program currently provide training on taking a sexual history as part of geriatric education? Please explain.
(2) What barriers have you experienced in addressing older adult sexuality and sexual history taking in geriatric training?
(3) What resources would be useful to you in addressing older adult sexuality and sexual history taking in your geriatric program?

The recording of the focus group session was transcribed using voice recognition software, which was reviewed and corrected by two of the authors.

Quantitative measures

Geriatrics fellows were asked to complete a brief, structured questionnaire which contained the pre- and posttest items. Seven items assessed knowledge of sexual health issues in older adults and employed true/false and multiple choice response formats (see Table 1 for items). Scoring was based on the number of correct answers, with a possible range of 0 to 7. These items were adapted from materials previously developed from a training module on older adult sexuality conducted by ACRIA, which had been previously used successfully with health and social service providers. Three items assessed attitudes toward addressing sexual health with older patients using a Likert-type format on a 5-point scale (*strongly agree* to *strongly disagree*; see Table 1 for items). Additionally, four questions were asked about current sexual history taking practice prior to the skills-building session using a Likert-type format on a 5-point scale (*strongly agree* to *strongly disagree*; see Table 2 for items). Attitude and practice items were developed through discussions with members of the Consortium Planning Committee and were not pilot tested. At the end of the plenary session, posttest questionnaires were administered to assess the extent to which the training may have increased knowledge and self-efficacy concerning sexual history taking. Changes in the combined knowledge scores from pretest to posttest were examined using an independent sample t test. Significant changes at the item level between pre- and posttest were examined using Fisher's Exact Test.

Qualitative data

The transcription of the focus group was imported into qualitative analysis software program Atlas/ti (Muhr, 1997). A content analysis of these data was initially conducted by two

Table 1. Pre- and posttest results from Geriatrics Fellows Conference on Older Adult Sexuality.

Knowledge Items	Pretest		Posttest		p Value
	n	%	n	%	
After the age of 60, older adults are not sexually active.					
True	0	0.0	1	2.9	
False[a]	28	100.0	33	97.1	1.00
Older women are most likely to be sexually inactive because of:					
Poor general health	5	18.5	3	9.1	
Not having a sexual partner[a]	18	66.7	28	84.9	
Lack of interest in sex	3	11.1	2	6.0	
Inability to climax	1	3.7	0	0.0	.33
Older men are most likely to be sexually inactive because of:					
Poor general health[a]	15	53.6	17	50.0	
Not having a sexual partner	7	25.0	3	8.8	
Lack of interest in sex	0	0.0	0	0.0	
Inability to climax	6	21.4	14	41.2	.11
Sex for the older adult may focus more on kissing/hugging as a means of intimacy as compared with genital contact or intercourse.					
True[a]	20	71.4	30	88.2	
False	8	28.6	4	11.8	.12
What proportion of older adults have talked with their physicians about sex after age 50?					
100%	0	0.0	0	0.0	
75%	1	3.6	0	0.0	
50%	3	10.7	1	2.9	
Less than 50%[a]	24	85.7	33	97.1	.21
Older women are at increased risk for sexually transmitted infections due to thinning of the vaginal walls and poor lubrication.					
True[a]	21	75.0	28	82.4	
False	7	25.0	6	17.7	.54
Erectile dysfunction medications has been related to an increase in sexually transmitted infections in older men.					
True[a]	12	42.9	32	94.1	
False	16	57.1	2	5.9	.001

Attitude Items	Pretest		Posttest		p Value
	n	%	n	%	
I am less likely to take a sexual history if my patient is…					
Older than me	9	33.3	14	41.2	
Different racial/ethnic background than me	1	11.1	5	15.2	
Different gender than me	9	34.6	12	35.3	
Different sexual orientation than me	3	12.5	6	18.2	.77
Sexual health is a more important component of overall physical and mental health for younger adults compared to older adults.					
Strongly agree	2	7.1	2	5.9	
Agree	6	21.4	9	26.5	
Neither agree nor disagree	8	28.6	5	14.7	
Disagree	9	32.1	14	41.2	
Strongly disagree	3	10.7	4	11.8	.75
I am confident about my ability to take a sexual history with my older patients.					
Strongly agree	0	0	5	15.2	
Agree	12	42.9	15	45.5	
Neither agree nor disagree	10	35.7	9	27.3	
Disagree	5	17.9	4	12.1	
Strongly disagree	1	3.6	0	0	.18

Note. Pre-test N = 28; Post-test N = 34.
a. Correct items for knowledge.

researchers not present during the focus group using an inductive process with open coding. This initial analysis was reviewed by the focus group facilitator with the two researchers, and the preliminary findings were harmonized through discussion. The harmonized content analysis was shared with the Consortium Project Planning Committee to provide feedback

Table 2. Sexual health and history practice items.

Item	n	%
How often do you collect a sexual history from your older adult patients?		
All of the time	2	7.1
Some of the time	7	25.0
Only occasionally	15	53.6
Not at all	4	14.3
How often do you update an older patient's sexual history?		
At every visit	1	3.6
Annually	3	10.7
If the patient's condition changes	8	28.6
Infrequently or never	16	57.1
How often do you discuss factors for sexually transmitted infections with older patients?		
All of the time	0	0.0
Some of the time	5	17.9
Only occasionally	12	42.9
Not at All	11	39.3
I am more comfortable with taking a sexual history from an older patient after attending today's symposium.		
Strongly agree	9	26.5
Agree	23	67.7
Neither agree nor disagree	1	2.9
Disagree	1	2.9
Strongly disagree	0	0.0

and corroborate the findings. The Project Planning Committee provided additional comments to the researchers to resolve any disagreement concerning content and interpretation in an iterative process. The transcript was corrected and reanalyzed based on this feedback and then reviewed and confirmed a final time by the Project Planning Committee.

Results

Quantitative findings

Sexual health knowledge

Overall, the geriatric fellows demonstrated that they were knowledgeable about older adult sexuality, and only one of the knowledge items showed any significant change between pre- and posttest (see Table 1). The only question that demonstrated statistically significant change at the item level was whether erectile dysfunction medications were related to greater incidence of STIs in older men, increasing from 43% correct at pretest to 94% at posttest. However, the summary score of correct answers on the knowledge questions did significantly increase from a mean of 4.96 (SD = 1.3) at pr-test to 6.00 (SD = .94) at posttest, $t(48)$ = 3.66, p < .001, which indicates that overall, geriatric fellows' knowledge of older adult sexuality increased after attending the psychosocial plenary presentation.

Attitude items

On the three attitude items, no significant differences between pre- and posttest at the item level were observed. With regard to patient characteristics that would inhibit taking a sexual history, the two most frequently endorsed responses (approximately one third of respondents) were if the patient is "older than me" and if the patient is a "different gender than me." Approximately one-in-10 felt that differences in racial/ethnic background was a deterrent to taking a sexual history whereas about one-in-six would have been inhibited if the patient was of a different sexual orientation. With regard to the statement that sexual health is a more important issue for younger as opposed to older adults, 43% indicated *disagree/strongly disagree* at pretest, which rose to 53% *disagree/strongly disagree* at posttest. However, this change was not statistically significant. In terms of the final attitude question about if they were confident in taking a sexual history with older adults, 43% of fellows agreed with the statement at pretest (no one strongly agreed), which rose to 61% agree/strongly agree at posttest, but this change was not statistically significant (see Table 1).

Practice items

Table 2 shows the results of the four questions about current sexual history taking practices among the geriatric fellows at the conference. With regard to sexual history taking with older adult patients, 14% reported "never" taking sexual histories whereas a majority (54%) said they did so "only occasionally." One fourth said they took sexual histories from older adults "some of the time" and 7% (*n* = 2) indicated that they always engaged in this practice. However, even when sexual histories were taken with older adult patients, this information was rarely updated in a systematic manner. Only one geriatric fellow indicated updating sexual history information at every visit (4%), whereas 11% of fellows updated sexual histories annually. Approximately 29% of fellows updated sexual histories if the condition of their older patient changed, but 57% reported they updated these histories "infrequently or never."

Responses to the frequency of discussing risks for STIs with older patients reflected the low rate of taking sexual histories, with none of the fellows reporting they did this "all of the time" and 18% saying these discussions were engaged in "some of the time." Additionally, 43% reported having STI risk discussions with older patients "only occasionally," and a nearly equal proportion (39%) did not have these discussions with older patients. When asked if attendance at the day's psychosocial conference on older adult sexuality had made them feel more comfortable with the idea of taking a sexual history from an older patient, 94% agreed or strongly agreed with that statement. This finding suggests that continuing education on the topic of sex and older adults could be useful in increasing the rate of sexual history taking in this population.

Qualitative findings

Qualitative data from the focus group of geriatric program directors, faculty, and other health professionals were obtained to have a better understanding of the current level of knowledge, attitudes, and practice concerning sexual health issues in older adults observed in the geriatric fellows attending the psychosocial conference. These data also helped to identify gaps and development needs for sexual health content in geriatric curricula. The information from this session is presented within the context of the three questions that framed this discussion.

(1) Does your fellowship program currently provide training on taking a sexual history as part of geriatric education? Please explain.

Only three out of 28 individuals indicated that their fellowship programs currently addressed taking a sexual history as part of their school's geriatric curriculum. In the discussion that followed, it became clear that older adult sexual health, even when included, was not a major component of the curriculum, even though most endorsed the importance of this topic based on their clinical experience. One person related the situation of many older women who find themselves single, either from being widowed or divorced, and new to the dating scene. She went on to say that because they were postmenopausal, there was an enhanced enjoyment of sex for these women. Without pregnancy concerns, condoms and other STI prevention methods were rarely employed. Another person described her experience with older men having multiple partners that increases the risk of STIs, as well as situation where one spouse may have dementia whereas the other spouse desires to remain sexually active. She explained that the latter situation is further complicated with the presence of adult children who might discover their parent is having sex outside of the marital relationship due to the illness of the spouse.

A number of participants identified specific needs around improving expertise and knowledge around older adult sexual health, including skills building, practical training, observation in taking a sexual history, and role-playing. One participant described the situation at her institution where one of the instructors provided a one-hour lecture on sexual health and how to deal with uncomfortable situations, which though helpful, did not fully address training needs:

> It is not a workshop so certainly it would be better if we observed them [the fellows] doing this but at least it is provided with this lecture and sometimes it's incorporated in one of our case conferences, which may or may not happen yearly.

Sexual health issues were addressed in geriatric curricula in other nonsystematic ways. One person described how his or her journal club sometimes had articles relating to older adult sexuality that prompted a discussion on how to facilitate conversations with their older patients. In some instances, sexual health content was addressed due to the interests of geriatric faculty who might choose to give a lecture on the topic, or due to their professional interest on a topic related to sexual health (e.g., HIV and older adults), or because they recently treated a patient who had a sexual health issue.

It was clear that this discussion was provoking a lot of thought on the part of participants regarding how they could address sexual health needs of older adults in geriatric education. One person shared that she had received a grant in the past to develop a geriatric curriculum for the American College of Obstetrics and Gynecology (OBGYN). In seeking creative ways to engage OBGYN physicians on a topic that they might have great interest (geriatrics), her team constructed a series of computer games and interactive computer modules including a video. She believed that these materials could be readily adapted for geriatric education.

(2) What barriers have you experienced in addressing older adult sexuality and sexual history taking in geriatric training?

Two major issues emerged as barriers to addressing the sexual health needs of older adults: competition with other geriatric core competencies and lack of educational resources. With regard to the former, one participant noted the list of 76 curriculum competencies in geriatrics that drive geriatric education and do not include sexual health (Parks, Harper, Fernandez, Sauvigne, & Leipzig, 2014). This person stated:

> I do not think it is a lack of being informed but there's so many other things that are important, at least for us, and now I realize that actually doing this for the past few months,

actually concentrating on the sexual history, how we are missing a component, although it is not listed in the curriculum, it is still important.

There was also the idea that if sexual health could not be addressed in the standard geriatric curriculum, there were other mechanisms in which to address the topic. One person noted that her institution had a psychosocial monthly meeting with the geriatrics fellows on various topics, and that older adult sexual health information could be included in that setting.

In addition to competing curricular demands, an important consideration was the readiness of geriatric faculty to address sexual health and older adults. One participant noted, "[We] need to make faculty more comfortable discussing sexual histories with geriatric patients and teaching it at medical schools." Related to this was the observation by many of the participants that education regarding human sexuality was frequently handled by nonphysician faculty at medical schools, namely, social workers and psychologists. Although some institutions did address psychosocial issues without having nonmedical faculty, this did create a barrier. One person stated, "So it would typically be a social worker that would provide this—I'm not sure most programs have a social worker, psychologist or psychiatrist."

(3) What resources would be useful to you in addressing older adult sexuality and sexual history taking in your geriatric program?

One respondent stated that an important resource was additional interdisciplinary faculty who could be called upon to address specific patient problems, in this case, sexual health. These individuals could be accessed to help develop a geriatric sexual health curriculum. There were specific content areas within the domain of sexual health that were identified as being crucial. One was sexual activity for patients with dementia, their spouses/partners, and the patients' family. Another person emphasized the need to consider all of the ramifications of sexual activity in curriculum development:

Also, I think it's important for there to be some information about the connection between sexuality, sexual assault and sexual rights, so when people are developing curriculum, it is just a way of bringing in ... how those issues can be connected.

One participant noted the need for specific knowledge and training around sexual orientation and gender diversity in older adults given their unique needs and the need to approach sexual health matters in a sensitive manner with these communities. She noted that her institution has facilities in a neighborhood with a large population of lesbian, gay, bisexual, and transgender older adults (LGBT). She also felt that given the disproportionate impact of HIV/AIDS in LGBT communities and the greying of this population, more information was needed on HIV and aging given the growing concentration of older adults with this condition in clinical settings.

Discussion

Although fairly knowledgeable about older adult sexuality, geriatrics fellows' knowledge scale scores increased significantly following the plenary presentation. Thus, it appears that this group of professionals would benefit from timely educational programs addressing older adult sexuality. These programs could be incorporated into geriatrics curriculum and continuing education opportunities. Despite this level of knowledge among these geriatricians, taking sexual histories and updating such histories with older patients was infrequent. Although attitudes towards taking sexual histories did not change as the result of the plenary session, responses to the item on barriers to taking sexual histories among older patients were most strongly related to provider-patient differences with regard to age and gender. Because geriatrics fellows reported greater confidence in taking sexual histories following the skills-building session, the inclusion of this type of educational activity in geriatrics curricula could greatly improve attention to the sexual health needs of older patients.

The need for sexual health education was recognized by the fellows, program directors, faculty, and other health professionals as an important component in geriatric clinical care but often not included in the curriculum. Clinically competent care in conducting a sexual history is needed for physicians at all levels of experience. To address this gap, a multidisciplinary approach is needed to create educational materials and curriculum. There were very few case scenarios in the literature review that addressed the kind of complex formative teaching or evaluations needed for geriatrics fellowship curricula.

Implications for geriatrics education and training

It is clear from the plenary and focus group session that further fellowship curriculum development is warranted, as well as continued research on the heterogeneity of the geriatric population and the intersection of medical care and sexual health. Some methods to achieve this are:

- Increased awareness: Emphasizing knowledge of the facts of sexuality in older adults and the need for incorporating sexual histories into routine geriatric practice while taking cultural difference into consideration is needed.
- Expand available educational tools: Develop new materials and identify nursing, social work and other disciplines with existing curricula that can be used by geriatrics fellowship programs. One example would be a video interview with an older woman describing to her physician her active sexual feelings and her loss of her long-term partner.
- Greater partnerships with community and other health care providers: Since nurses, social workers, therapists, urologists, and gynecologists in medical and community setting are often managing patients with sexual problems, these colleagues are an important source of educational and clinical support for geriatrics programs. Such partnerships could be a particularly valuable resource for geriatrics programs that do not have ready resources to provide in-house training on older adult sexuality.
- Foster stronger connections to LGBT and other special needs communities: It is important to address LGBT sexuality issues throughout a patient's life span. Collaboration of faculty and trainees with interdisciplinary community resources is essential in responding to the multifaceted needs of these and other marginalized groups.
- Improved awareness of victims of elder abuse: Recognizing that sexual abuse occurs in older adults and may become apparent in clinical settings is key in the identification, assessment, and provision of appropriate interventions.
- Increased comfort level around sexual health topics for faculty in practice and in teaching: We need a better understanding of faculty's comfort level and how this may have an impact on teaching and practice. Faculty should explore ways to overcome barriers to addressing patients' sexual health and augment clinical skills to improve practice.

Limitations

The findings from this article are limited due to the small sample of geriatrics fellows from urban areas of the northeastern United States that may limit generalizability because of regional differences in attitudes towards older adult sexuality. However, the data presented here are consistent with other published work and can serve as a springboard to addressing older adult sexual health in a larger context. In addition, because there was no comparison group for the knowledge pre- and posttests, we cannot be certain if the gains in knowledge scores were the result of attending the plenary educational session or were the result of testing effects.

Conclusions

Due to the failure of health care providers in general to address sexual health needs in older patients, the focus of this article is to address this gap in geriatrics sexual health education. Geriatricians and other health care providers reflect our larger society and the myths and misunderstandings in our culture regarding aging and sexuality (Dominguez & Barbagallo, 2016). Because health care providers and older adults themselves have difficulties discussing sexual matters in clinical settings (Hughes & Lewinson, 2015), it is imperative to help providers foster communication by encouraging patients to share their sexual lives, building trust, and establishing rapport with their older patients (Hughes & Lewinson, 2015).

Part of the solution to this need lies in professional education and preparation. In a review of graduate nursing programs, Musumeci-Szabo and Thomas-Cottingham (2016) found that though many programs offered tracks or programs in gerontology, very few addressed sexual health among older adults. In a survey of 278 physicians and nurses in primary care, 11% felt their training on older adult sexuality was adequate and only 3% felt they had adequate knowledge of the topic (Hughes & Wittmann, 2015). Thus, the need to expand training and education efforts for medical and nonmedical providers across disciplines is vital. Existing training and education efforts around older adult sexuality have been found to be effective in increasing knowledge and improving practice in the domains of long-term care (Mayers & McBride, 1998), residential care (Bauer, McAulliffe, Nay, & Chenco, 2013), LGBT sexuality (Hardacker, Rubinstein, Hotton, & Houlberg, 2014), psychology (Gray-Miceli et al., 2014), and senior services (Seidel, Karpiak, & Brennan-Ing, 2017). These successful training programs could serve as a model for improving older adult sexuality training in geriatrics education and improve sexual health care for our aging population.

References

Adelman, R. D., Ansell, P., Breckman, R., Snow, C. E., Ehrlich, A. R., Greene, M. G., ... Fields, S. D. (2011). Building psychosocial programming in geriatrics fellowships: A consortium model. *Gerontology & Geriatrics Education*, *32*(4), 309–320. doi:10.1080/02701960.2011.611558

Alexander, S. C., Fortenberry, J. D., Pollak, K. I., Bravender, T., Davis, J. K., Østbye, T., ... Shields, C. G. (2014). Sexuality talk during adolescent health maintenance visits. *JAMA Pediatrics*, *168*(2), 163–169. doi:10.1001/jamapediatrics.2013.4338

Amin, I. (2016). Social capital and sexual risk-taking behaviors among older adults in the United States. *Journal of Applied Gerontology*, *35*(9), 982–999. doi:10.1177/0733464814547048

Bauer, M., McAuliffe, L., Nay, R., & Chenco, C. (2013). Sexuality in older adults: Effect of an education intervention on attitudes and beliefs of residential aged care staff. *Educational Gerontology, 39*(2), 82–91. doi:10.1080/03601277.2012.682953

Dominguez, L. J., & Barbagallo, M. (2016). Ageing and sexuality. *European Geriatric Medicine, 7,* 512–518. doi:10.1016/j.eurger.2016.05.013

Golub, S. A., Tomassilli, J. C., Pantalone, D. W., Brennan, M., Karpiak, S. E., & Parsons, J. T. (2010). Prevalence and correlates of sexual behavior and risk management among HIV-positive adults over 50. *Sexually Transmitted Diseases, 37*(10), 615–620.

Gray-Miceli, D., Wilson, L. D., Stanley, J., Watman, R., Shire, A., Sofaer, S., & Mezey, M. (2014). Improving the quality of geriatric nursing care: Enduring outcomes from the Geriatric Nursing Education Consortium. *Journal of Professional Nursing, 30*(6), 447–455. doi:10.1016/j.profnurs.2014.05.001

Hardacker, C. T., Rubinstein, B., Hotton, A., & Houlberg, M. (2014). Adding silver to the rainbow: The development of the nurses' health education about LGBT elders (HEALE) cultural competency curriculum. *Journal of Nursing Management, 22*(2), 257–266. doi:10.1111/jonm.2014.22.issue-2

Hughes, A. K., & Lewinson, T. D. (2015). Facilitating communication about sexual health between aging women and their health care providers. *Qualitative health research, 25*(4), 540–550.

Hughes, A. K., Rostant, O. S., & Pelon, S. (2015). Sexual problems among older women by age and race. *Journal of Women's Health, 24*(8), 663–669. doi:10.1089/jwh.2014.5010

Hughes, A. K., & Wittmann, D. (2015). Aging sexuality: Knowledge and perceptions of preparation among US primary care providers. *Journal of Sex & Marital Therapy, 41*(3), 304–313. doi:10.1080/0092623X.2014.889056

Lindau, S. T., Schumm, L. P., Laumann, E. O., Levinson, W., O'Muircheartaigh, C. A., & Waite, L. J. (2007). A study of sexuality and health among older adults in the United States. *New England Journal of Medicine, 357*(8), 762–774. doi:10.1056/NEJMoa067423

Liu, H., Waite, L., Shen, S., & Wang, D. (2016). Is sex good for your health? A national study on partnered sexuality and cardiovascular risk among older men and women. *Journal of Health and Social Behavior, 57*(3), 276–296. doi:10.1177/0022146516661597

Marsiglio, W., & Donnelly, D. (1991). Sexual relations in later life: A national study of married persons. *Journal of Gerontology, 46*(6), S338–S344. doi:10.1093/geronj/46.6.S338

Mayers, K. S., & McBride, D. (1998). Sexuality training for caretakers of geriatric residents in long term care facilities. *Sexuality and Disability, 16*(3), 227–236. doi:10.1023/A:1023003310885

Milrod, C., & Monto, M. (2016). Older male clients of female sex workers in the United States. *Archives of Sexual Behavior,* 1–10.

Minkin, M. J. (2016). Sexual health and relationships after age 60. *Maturitas, 83,* 27–32. doi:10.1016/j.maturitas.2015.10.004

Muhr, T. (1997). Atlas/ti for Windows: Visual qualitative data analysis, management, & model building [computer software]. Berlin: Scientific Software Development.

Musumeci-Szabo, T. J., & Thomas-Cottingham, A. (2016, November). *You can't teach what you don't know: Sexual health and aging in graduate nursing curriculum.* Poster presentation at the 69th Annual Scientific Meeting of the Gerontological Society of America, New Orleans, LA.

Parks, S. M., Harper, G. M., Fernandez, H., Sauvigne, K., & Leipzig, R. M. (2014). American geriatrics society/association of directors of geriatric academic programs curricular milestones for graduating geriatric fellows. *Journal of the American Geriatrics Society, 62*(5), 930–935. doi:10.1111/jgs.12821

Patel, D., Gillespie, B., & Foxman, B. (2003). Sexual behavior of older women: Results of a random-digit-dialing survey of 2000 women in the United States. *Sexually Transmitted Diseases, 30*(3), 216–220. doi:10.1097/00007435-200303000-00008

Pera, A., Campos, C., López, N., Hassouneh, F., Alonso, C., Tarazona, R., & Solana, R. (2015). Immunosenescence: Implications for response to infection and vaccination in older people. *Maturitas, 82*(1), 50–55. doi:10.1016/j.maturitas.2015.05.004

Reece, M., Herbenick, D., Schick, V., Sanders, S. A., Dodge, B., & Fortenberry, J. D. (2010). Condom use rates in a national probability sample of males and females ages 14 to 94 in the United States. *Journal of Sexual Medicine, 7*(s5), 266–276. doi:10.1111/j.1743-6109.2010.02017.x

Schick, V., Herbenick, D., Reece, M., Sanders, S. A., Dodge, B., Middlestadt, S. E., & Fortenberry, J. D. (2010). Sexual behaviors, condom use, and sexual health of Americans over 50: Implications for sexual health promotion for older adults. *Journal of Sexual Medicine*, *7*(s5), 315–329. doi:10.1111/j.1743-6109.2010.02013.x

Seidel, L., Karpiak, S. E., & Brennan-Ing, M. (2017). Training senior service providers about HIV and Aging: Evaluation of a Multi-year, Multi-City Initiative. *Gerontology and Geriatrics Education*, *38*(2), 188–203. DOI:10.1080/02701960.2015.1090293

Smith, K. P., & Christakis, N. A. (2009). Association between widowhood and risk of diagnosis with a sexually transmitted infection in older adults. *American Journal of Public Health*, *99*(11), 2055–2062. doi:10.2105/AJPH.2009.160119

Index